Praise for
Surviving Healthcare in Australia

The Australian Healthcare system has the potential to be world-class but is undermined by complexity, incongruity and a lack of systemic coordination. There is a need for patient-centric, holistic, value healthcare. In *Surviving Healthcare in Australia: Get the Support You Need*, Anne Crawford draws on her own extensive experience to provide insights and valuable tips on how everyday Australians can navigate the healthcare system to access better care and how our system can be improved to fulfil its potential.

Dr. Elizabeth Sigston
MBBS FRACS PhD

Surviving Healthcare in Australia is a 'must read' if you want to know about the support and care options available to you. Patient care doesn't have to be one dimensional, as it sometimes seems!

Rachel Johnson
Founder of HAAA and wSw

Overall, this book is a great introduction to the history and complexity of Australia's healthcare system, while introducing us to a potential solution or mechanism that will make this journey simpler.

Tom Voigt
Senior Policy & Research Officer,
Australian Association of Gerontology (AAG)

Anne Crawford's book demonstrates the need for modern approaches to remove the complexity that exists today in our healthcare system and restore trust back into the community. It highlights the importance for putting patients and their families at the centre of decisions and working alongside healthcare professionals to get the best possible outcome. *Surviving Healthcare in Australia* is a great book.

Paul Montgomery
Chair, MediSecure Limited and Wellways Australia,
Director, Melbourne Primary Care Network

SURVIVING HEALTHCARE IN AUSTRALIA

Get the Support You Need

■ SECOND EDITION ■

SURVIVING HEALTHCARE IN AUSTRALIA

Get the Support You Need

SECOND EDITION

ANNE CRAWFORD, MPH

Foreword by Felicity Smith OAM

EMERALD LAKE
BOOKS
Sherman, Connecticut

Surviving Healthcare in Australia: Get the Support You Need
Second Edition

Copyright © 2023 Anne Crawford

Cover design by Mark Gerber

Books published by Emerald Lake Books may be ordered through your favorite booksellers or by visiting emeraldlakebooks.com.

ISBN: 978-1-945847-52-3 (paperback)
        978-1-945847-53-0 (epub)
        978-1-945847-54-7 (large print)

Library of Congress Control Number: 2022901869

This book is dedicated to:

My husband and daughter.
I have always wanted to write this book and they
are the reason I have been able to. My husband
has been my anchor, my partner, friend and mentor.
My daughter has been my inspiration for this topic.

My ever-loving parents.
They have always been there for me
and supported my development.

Contents

Foreword

As a population, the health and health experiences of Australians compare well with those of other countries. And our life expectancy at birth remains among the highest in the world.

However, Australia's healthcare system is striving for efficiency. As a result, busy health professionals may tend to treat patient conditions solely on the basis of symptoms and scientific evidence. Unfortunately, this can lead to a reduced consideration of the patient as a person, who may be suffering from more than one condition or have other factors that should be taken into account before settling on a treatment plan.

The Australian health system is often too complicated for patients to navigate on their own. This issue is amplified by an ageing population and the anticipated rise in chronic disease. Therefore, we need to strengthen primary healthcare to better co-ordinate the care of patients and decrease the risk of medical errors that are unacceptable to patients and costly for everyone.

When health professionals, patients, families and carers work in partnership, the quality and safety of healthcare improves, costs decrease, provider satisfaction increases, and the patient care experience is enhanced.

This book draws on Anne's experience as an industry healthcare professional, as well as being a patient and a carer for a child with a severe disability. It provides a compelling solution to improve a complicated system and is worthy of discussion well into the future. This book will present any reader with great insight into what is missing in the healthcare system.

I have known the author for a many years and am intimately acquainted the challenges she has faced. As Anne has dealt with each of these issues, she has always looked for ways to make things better.

As a mother of three adult sons with their own particular health issues, I too have dealt with my own challenges within the Australian healthcare system. Navigating a system that seems more intent on refusing you help when you most need it has been difficult and disheartening for me.

I commend the dedication of her determination in preparing this book, and highly recommend reading it.

Felicity Smith OAM
Chair, Board of Directors
Link Health & Community

Introduction

Healthcare systems around the world are constantly changing and developing, dependent on costs and demands like any service industry. In Australia, we have a world-class healthcare system, Medicare, that is the envy of most of the developed world. But it is still very confusing and inaccessible.

By profession, I am a nurse and midwife, and I have earned my Master's degree in Public Health. I have also worked in hospitals, aged care homes and in the community alongside general practitioners. I am currently on the board of several community health services. So, I have an intimate knowledge of Australia's healthcare system from a professional perspective.

However, I also have extensive experience with it from a personal standpoint. As a young adult, I cared for my grandmother in her final years, and I now have a daughter with special needs. In addition, a number of years ago, my eyes were injured in an accident and I came to experience how rare it is for our healthcare system to work to its full potential.

This exposure as a medical professional, patient and caregiver has provided me with an intimate understanding of how our healthcare system is supposed to work.

In writing this book, I am motivated by the following concern: *If I can't negotiate my way around the healthcare system (despite my extensive education, experience and knowledge), how does anyone else do it?*

As you read, you will discover that this book is purposely not academic in nature. In it, I use real case studies to illustrate what can go wrong in healthcare and why.[1] Yet each story ends on a positive note and shares key points you can use to help you manage your own way through the healthcare system in Australia.

My hope is to convey some ideas about how to navigate through the system, as well as to provide an overview of where we have come from and how the system works today. Finally, I will provide some possible solutions to the current inequalities and frustrations that people experience.

While this book is intended for people who are currently going through diagnosis and treatment, or who are supporting a loved one with a health crisis, it is also relevant for lawmakers and policy changers. As world-class as our healthcare system is, there is still room (and need) for improvement.

The current system must begin to provide more well-rounded (or holistic) care for people and to acknowledge patients as the decision makers about their own treatment and ongoing care.

This approach requires that healthcare providers share enough appropriate information and guidance for their patients to make informed decisions. However, our current healthcare model works on

---

1   Details and names have been changed to maintain privacy.

the premise that the treating provider is the one who knows what is needed for the individual. This book challenges that viewpoint.

Although healthcare providers are starting to talk about partnering with patients, these professionals must understand that patients are not partners—healthcare professionals do not share in the problems these individuals are facing. There is no impact on the life of a healthcare provider when a patient is sick, except that it provides them with a job.

For example, if a patient requires surgery followed by a six-week recovery, the surgeon does not have to cope with the pain or manage home affairs while the patient is recovering. The surgeon performs the surgery and then prescribes the medication he or she believes the patient needs. The surgeon may suggest physiotherapy to ensure the recovery is as efficient as it can be, but it is the patient who is left to deal with the whole picture.

It is time that our healthcare system provides patients with the support they need, not just to recover from an illness, but to secure the best possible outcome physically, mentally, emotionally *and* personally.

Chapter One

The Missing Ingredient
in Our Healthcare System

Healthcare in Australia is world-class and we are able to boast about equity and access. While we do have problems with access in our more remote regions, we have a fair system that caters well for most people. So why do people find the healthcare system so inhospitable and frustrating? If they are lucky, they will find support services by chance or word of mouth. But why is the system so confusing and why don't healthcare providers seem to know what is available for the community they support?

In my professional capacity, I am regularly asked how to access support services. Many people in our community do not know what is available to help them manage at home during an illness. There are also many people who don't know what to do when they are sick.

The health service system has become so specialised that there are practitioners who don't really understand how to help people outside their scope of knowledge. But people are not just a medical illness. They are breadwinners, parents, children, siblings, partners or active members of their community. This means that when they fall ill, they need more than just medicine. They need a whole support system to get back to being themselves.

I have been to meetings of parents with disabled teenagers who did not know anything about support services for their children except for attending a special school. The families had missed out on so much. They were under financial strain that was causing tension in their partnership, and it could have been avoided had they known more about the services available to them.

There are many people in our country who struggle with mental health issues, alcohol and drug addiction, homelessness and social isolation. We are a rich country, but we still have many people who are struggling. And healthcare practitioners have become so specialised that they can miss the whole picture. We have made our healthcare system so complex and inaccessible that people often feel confused and unheard, and think their concerns are not being dealt with.

Australia's healthcare system has developed organically, beginning largely as charity or a service to those who could afford it. If people were sick and poor, they had to rely on charity or their families to act as carers. Many people went bankrupt trying to pay for their healthcare. Now we have a system that is capable of providing so much to the people it supports, if they only knew how to access those services.

When Australia entered the World Wars as part of the Commonwealth, it improved how healthcare was delivered. Most hospitals trained staff as if they were part of the army. It was very regimented, and patients and staff were designated into wards that became specialised in the areas of the body that were being treated.

Medical staff grew proficient in the treatment and care of people's illnesses. Research into healthcare also became specialised. Treatments improved, and hospitals became centres of healthcare excellence.

This evolution explains how gaps in healthcare began to develop—each specialty became adept at managing certain conditions but lost sight of the whole picture. As knowledge and complexity developed, the gaps grew.[2]

We have a healthcare system that considers itself the 'holder of special knowledge'. Healthcare providers believe they are the experts and should be the ones making decisions about the person they are caring for. However, although healthcare providers do have specialised knowledge, they may not know a person's particular circumstances and may not consider the implications of treatment options on that person's life.

Decisions about treatment should essentially be left up to the individuals themselves. They need to be the ones who make the final decision about whether to go ahead with a treatment that has been offered.

---

2   To learn more about the history of this evolution, read 'Appendix: A Short History of the Australian Healthcare System' page 141.

There are many areas in the healthcare system where people are likely to fall through the gaps. Not having an understanding of the support they require or how to access such support means that people are being left to manage on their own. This puts them at risk of returning to the doctor or the hospital because they did not understand what they were supposed to do or what support they could access for help.

We have new ways to fund the Australian health system that have caused anxiety for both the patient and service providers. For example, the disability sector is transitioning to the National Disability Insurance Scheme (NDIS) and the aged care sector has recently transitioned to a similar scheme called 'My Aged Care'. Although there are many benefits to these changes, it has made an already confusing system even worse for both patients and healthcare professionals alike.

Dental care has never been well-funded by the federal government and is largely supported by state and territory systems. This has led to people simply not being able to access dental care, or having exceedingly long wait times to see a public dentist.

Finally, what happens when a patient goes to a doctor with a health complaint and there is no clear diagnosis? The healthcare professional will often label the person as a 'malingerer'. Thus, a person who complains when the healthcare provider cannot provide an identifiable answer is considered either psychologically impaired, lying or both.

In my experience, it is uncommon for the medical profession to acknowledge that medicine still has a long way to go in identifying many of the different conditions that can affect people. Instead, someone with an undiagnosed illness is often sent away feeling confused and unsupported. They become disillusioned and frustrated after being treated as if they are 'putting on' their symptoms, and it often has an impact on their personal relationships and ability to work.

Instead, the healthcare provider needs to consider the limitations of assessments and medical tests, and listen to the person's concerns. If there is an ongoing health issue, treatment of the symptoms may be the best solution, even if the condition itself cannot be identified. This requires a deep knowledge of the treatment services available. Since the Australian healthcare system is so complex, this can be a challenge for any healthcare provider.

Olive's journey through pain management.

'Olive' (as we shall call her) went to see her general practitioner (GP). She had many medical issues and was often mismanaged since her medical conditions interacted with each other. Olive had developed a good relationship with her GP over many years, and he was aware that Olive's many conditions interact negatively.

One day, she was in significant pain. She had injured her shoulder and neck through repetitive and significant strain on her left arm at work. In addition, she felt pins and needles down her arm and had lost strength in her left hand. A scan showed mild herniations in two of the discs in her neck. Not wanting to miss anything, the GP sent her to the hospital for further assessment.

Olive arrived at the hospital with a letter from the GP, and she was quickly assessed by a young emergency doctor. He was also concerned and admitted her to the hospital.

While she was still in the emergency department, Olive had a respiratory allergic reaction. Her symptoms were unusual and looked like a severe asthma attack. (Her allergy symptoms were respiratory in nature, not the usual anaphylactic reaction many people experience.) Her husband, Chris, was with her and he gave her an EpiPen treatment, as he had been taught to do by her GP and allergy specialist. The emergency doctor was not happy that Chris had done this and told him so.

Eventually, Olive was admitted to the ward and was seen by the senior specialist. He ordered a few tests and gave her some pain medication. As is often the case with Olive, nothing appeared in the tests they administered. Olive knew that one of her specialists, a rheumatologist, had visiting rights at the hospital so she requested to see him. He did not come to see her during the admission and Olive was referred on for rehabilitation.

When Olive went to the rehabilitation centre, she was admitted by a doctor who specialised in pain management. This pain specialist never performed a physical examination of Olive, but he still organised her pain medication. During her stay, Olive was largely left to manage herself with little interaction with the medical staff, while the centre only provided her with a small amount of physiotherapy. Given the level of care she received, she likely would have been better off at home.

When she was discharged four weeks later, Olive felt no improvement and was groggy due to the medications she had been prescribed. She decided to see her rheumatologist for a review. The rheumatologist was exasperated because the medications prescribed by the pain specialist worked against Olive's rheumatology regimen.

He was also angry that no one had let him know about her admission. Despite many attempts by Olive and Chris, their messages had never reached him. He told Olive which medications he recommended she take, but decided against changing her prescriptions.

Olive had an appointment with the pain specialist she had seen in the rehabilitation centre for an outpatient review. She told him what the rheumatologist had recommended, and he changed her pain medications accordingly.

The pain specialist wrote a letter to her GP that speculated about the psychological states of Olive and her husband. He assumed a lot, as his assessment wasn't made in coordination with Olive or her husband. He had not performed any physical examinations and had not discussed any of his concerns with her. He inferred her pain was associated with psychological distress, despite the swelling in the area of concern. He suggested that her home life was stressful, and her husband was encouraging her to be unwell. (Olive's husband was understandably concerned about her, but he was not encouraging her in her 'sick role'.) The pain specialist questioned her allergy, because it did not have the usual signs associated with allergies (despite Olive's allergy specialist's assessment and diagnosis). He also doubted her willingness to rehabilitate, as she was so focused on her 'sick role'.

If the pain specialist had discussed any of his concerns or performed a physical examination of Olive, then his appraisal may have had some basis for believability. But he had simply read the notes in her file for this particular episode and taken other health professionals' assessments as adequate. He made no effort to contact her regular medical providers or learn more about her health history.

He was not helpful, and Olive spent four weeks convalescing in a rehabilitation centre when she could have used that time to heal and regain her physical strength.

On her last day in the hospital, Olive saw an inexperienced social worker and requested some help at home, but nothing was set up for her. Once she was home again, she became busy with her life. The social worker had given her a large bag of pamphlets, but they were too confusing, and Chris worked full-time and could not help her with more paperwork and phone calls.

Olive believed her time in hospital was not at all helpful, and that she had been left to figure out how to get better on her own. At home, she saw three different physiotherapists and continued to take her pain medications, which meant she could not drive. If she had to get to appointments, she had to rely on her family or take a taxi. It took six months for her to regain her strength and start to feel like her old self again.

She also saw her allergy specialist to discuss her allergy treatment, and he wrote a letter for Olive so that, if she went to hospital again, she could give them the letter for consistency of treatment. She did this because the hospital staff had not believed she had an allergy; instead they thought she was hyperventilating rather than having a reaction. Olive's immune system was so compromised, she had unusual signs and symptoms. Her immunologist was happy with her progress, however, so at least she did not have to receive additional treatment there.

Misdiagnosis, or a lack of diagnosis, and the impact it has on the patient.

Misdiagnosis happens a lot, as does a lack of diagnosis. This has an impact on a person's life and can affect their ability to work.

Olive's case study shows how those of us in the healthcare profession can miss important cues and make inadequate assessments when we use information from other providers. We are all human, and it is sometimes easy to copy others, which shortens the time spent gathering information. Unfortunately, if the information health professionals use is already tainted, the resulting diagnosis may be incorrect.

It is important for the health professional to assess people during their first meeting without relying on information gathered by others. Then if there is an inconsistency between their diagnosis and those of other medical professionals, it can be checked further.

I don't believe that Olive's case is necessarily a unique one, or that her doctors didn't care about what she was going through. But they each viewed her situation through the perspective of their speciality, rather than taking a holistic approach to her care and, in her case, that made her recovery more difficult than it needed to be.

Unfortunately, one of the most significant challenges that the medical profession faces is a lack of time to make a proper assessment of each individual case they may see. To spend the necessary time with them to get them to articulate their needs and provide the right support can be more than they can afford to give. It's not a matter of being uncaring or insensitive. They have a number of patients they must see, and simply lack suitable resources to take the necessary time.

For the healthcare system to work effectively, we need to ensure that GPs and other healthcare providers can refer their patients to a local community professional who has a deep knowledge of the health and community welfare services available to people, and who is dedicated to the special task of helping individuals navigate these challenging situations, not just physically, but mentally, emotionally and personally as well.

We shall call such a provider a 'healthcare coach' (or 'coach' for short). And while they can't be found in many communities yet, having such an individual available would make healthcare and its related services more accessible to those who need it most.

Right now, Australia has many different referral pathways (healthcare services, IT systems and web-based systems) to help people find services, but negotiating the healthcare system is complicated to those not familiar with it.

There are very experienced nurses who work in general practices or in the community (in other words, the Royal District Nursing Service or 'RDNS'), as well as local social workers and case managers. But unfortunately, they don't always have the training, experience or funding that allows them to spend the time required to provide the support individuals may need. Not because they don't want to, but because they may be limited by program parameters and, therefore, be unable to spend the time required to support patients until they are ready and able to manage their care on their own again.

Healthcare coaching is a role based on the concept of an executive coach, but for patients dealing with the healthcare system.

Medicare funds GPs, and also practice nurses in some instances, but there is no funding for a healthcare professional (or coach) who is adept at assessing a patient's requirements, and supporting and referring them appropriately. There have been projects periodically to support this process, but nothing to provide these experts with ongoing funding, either within a hospital system or associated with local GPs.

A solution could be to have healthcare coaches who are well-funded and resourced through Medicare working in both hospitals and the community. They could then support and direct people into appropriate individualised services.

These coaches may need to have a higher degree in nursing to be able to explain health conditions and their medications, and must have many years of relevant experience to bring to the role. Today, healthcare professionals suitably trained to act as a coach often end up in other roles, such as health service management, policy roles, research associates or consultants to people who can afford them.

This is despite the fact that having coaches available would reduce the waste and distress that comes with inappropriate referrals, or having people going in and out of hospital as a result of their condition not being adequately managed.

The problem with evidence-based practice.

Another issue that we, as medical professionals, have to deal with is that medical conditions affect people in different ways. We are trained to rely upon evidence-based research, which is typically conducted with otherwise healthy individuals, so the condition or treatment can be analysed in a regulated way. Gender differences are not considered, nor are cultural differences or people with more than one illness. Thus, although evidence-based medical or health decisions are the gold standard of care, they may not be the best option for a given individual.

Ideally, you should develop a relationship with your primary healthcare provider so they can take other needs and medical concerns into consideration when providing treatment options. The best healthcare professional to have an ongoing relationship with is your local general practitioner.

Chapter Two

The Role of the Primary Health Professional

Primary healthcare begins with seeing your general practitioner. Your local GP has extensive knowledge about many common medical conditions and can also provide guidance about your health and wellbeing. They are very competent and maintain their knowledge by reading current research about medical conditions as well as health and wellbeing. If you develop a long-term relationship with your GP, they can more easily identify medical problems that emerge.

Primary healthcare is healthcare that happens in the community. Ideally, we want to prevent health issues that land us in hospital since hospitals aren't good places to be. Prevention of health concerns begins with lifestyle (for example, eating well and doing regular exercise).

Ask your GP for advice on health management. A GP can discuss your issues and concerns regarding your health and assess your health status. They may refer you to a nutritionist, physiotherapist or other allied health professional for health maintenance. A

GP will also discuss vaccinations and monitoring for any familial medical conditions. Finally, they can also be very knowledgeable about stress management.

It is important to note that if you have not seen your GP for several years, then it has been too long. Why? Because there are health prevention activities that can be done to reduce the risk of worse things happening, including regular skin checks, pap smears and many other health checks. A GP who has a good working relationship with the local community health service can provide all the primary health management for you and your family.

Developing a relationship with your GP over time enables the GP to know when things change in your life.

Mary saw her GP over a two-year period.

Mary started seeing the GP because she was getting stomach pains. The only test that indicated anything was happening was her blood tests, which showed unusual liver test results. Often, that happens when the liver is inflamed. So, Mary was sent on a round of further tests and scans to see if the GP could identify why her liver was inflamed.

She was trying to have a child with her husband, so she was on medications for In Vitro Fertilisation (IVF). The IVF program requires that regular blood tests be taken. The GP could not find an answer to why her blood tests were showing an inflamed liver, so he sent her to a gastroenterologist who specialised in liver problems.

The specialist did several further tests, which included some exploratory surgery. During that time, the IVF program had to be postponed. After the surgery and testing, the specialist said she could not see any problems and therefore the specialist decided not to review Mary's case for three months.

Mary went back to the GP for a regular review and he was very concerned about one of the test results that had come back from the specialist. He then sent her to another gastro-enterologist.

The second specialist reviewed her test results and was very concerned. Mary had a cancerous growth in her gallbladder. This is a rare cancer, so it was fortunate that it was found early.

The whole family was really worried and came to help Mary and her husband. Mary had surgery and the new specialist was able to remove all the cancer. After her surgery, Mary was able to recommence her IVF. She requires regular screenings but has been free of cancer for five years.

Mary was fortunate that she had developed a relationship with her GP. It meant he was cautious and knew Mary often has problems that are not necessarily obvious. Without the conscientiousness of her GP, the cancer could have developed and become more serious.

Since then, Mary's liver tests have been fine. The GP continues to be conscientious and ensures Mary is seen regularly to check her health, refers her to exercise programs, and advises her on healthy eating habits.

After several tries at IVF, Mary had a healthy baby boy called 'James'.

General practitioners are your best medical advisers. The more you know them, the more they can help during a crisis.

Why a patient may prefer going to the local emergency department over seeing a GP.

The role of the GP in Australia is key in providing healthcare. A GP is able to monitor your condition and provide education about maintaining your health and wellbeing. It is necessary to understand though that, under our current healthcare system, it is cheaper and faster for patients to go to the emergency department than it is to go to a GP for a referral and then have tests and scans performed.

If a patient visits any public emergency department, everything is free of charge. The assessment is free. Any necessary tests are done immediately, also for free. If there is a medical concern, the patient is admitted into the hospital without delay.

If these services were done through the GP, it could take a week or more for the tests to be done, and most services have a co-payment, otherwise known as a 'gap fee' or 'out-of-pocket expense'. Then, if the patient needs to go to hospital, they have to wait again. So, from a patient's perspective, the decision is not just about cost, but also time spent waiting.

George kept visiting the local emergency department with minor ailments.

George had several chronic illnesses that he was managing at home. He lived with his wife, who was also unwell. He kept turning up at the local hospital emergency department every time he felt unwell. The RDNS was contacted by the hospital to help him with his medication regime and look at why he kept visiting the local hospital. Going to hospital is costlier to the Australian taxpayer than going to the local GP and it means that the emergency department beds are being taken up. This also results in ambulances having to go to another hospital with their emergency patients.

When the RDNS nurse, Sue, met with George, she could see that George and his wife were struggling to manage at home. Therefore, Sue provided further education to him about managing his medical conditions and she also set up some home support and Meals on Wheels. In addition, she got the pharmacist to organise their medication with a dosette pack, otherwise known as a 'Webster pack' or 'blister pack'.

By the time she was done, Sue believed that George and his wife would now be better supported and discharged them back to George's GP.

A month later, the local hospital's emergency department called Sue in again. She was worried that George and his wife might no longer be managing and that she would have to place them into aged care. Upon arriving at their home, however, she found them in a stable condition.

She asked George why he had gone to the hospital. He said, 'It's cheaper and faster for me to go to the hospital. I go to the hospital and I see the doctor and get tests done and it doesn't cost me anything. It's faster—the tests are done there.'

Sue explained to George and his wife why they needed to go to the local GP. She also spoke to the GP and the hospital about what she had found out from George.

George continued to go to the local hospital and they would send him to his GP for assessment.

After a few years, George and his wife moved in with their son and his family. The last time she visited, Sue found they were much happier. The son was building them a unit at the back of his home, and they appreciated the help that living near him would provide.

Medicare co-payments create a problem for healthcare professionals.

GPs are currently paid through Medicare and, for those people who can afford it, a co-payment. Often GPs will bulk-bill those who are pensioners or who have access to a Health Care Card, meaning that they waive the required co-payment. If you don't fit those categories, then there is an expectation that you will pay a portion of the service fees yourself.

If you can't afford the co-payment and are not a pensioner or don't have a Health Care Card, then you can speak to the GP about your financial concerns. A good GP will bulk-bill anyone experiencing financial distress. However, this negotiation must be done with the GP. The receptionist cannot make this decision.

But the co-payment makes up the smallest portion of the GP's payment. Medicare covers the rest once the appropriate information is filed about the patient's visit.

Each service listed on the Medicare Benefits Schedule (MBS) is assigned an item number, and a descriptor outlines the type and scope of the service and relevant clinical requirements.

In the initial stages of the Medicare system (in the 1980s), the MBS items that GPs could claim from the federal government included multiple kinds of clinical consultations. Commonly, GPs would conduct 15-minute consultations. This entitled them to claim the most common item number and collect their fees for the services they had provided. They often did this because it was a simple way to manage their claims.

Medicare claims were, and continue to be, audited regularly by the federal government. If the GP has not fulfilled all the criteria set in the MBS item number guidelines, they have to pay the money back. In the 1980s and 90s, this led to patients being rushed through their GP visits. At the time, it was disconcerting for the patients.

Now, MBS items number in the hundreds, which has made the system even more complicated. It means that GPs and specialists do not necessarily claim for services they provide. They find the system increasingly difficult to navigate and would prefer a simpler one. To help GPs manage, the federal government set up programs to educate them on how to more effectively use MBS item numbers. It is still very confusing, but GPs are getting better at knowing what they can claim.

Under the current funding scheme, Medicare only provides time for a GP to diagnose one condition at a time. If you have multiple concerns, you need to let the receptionist know in advance so they can book a longer appointment for you. The Medicare rebate is higher, but often so is the co-payment. If a longer appointment is required, it is often still cheaper and takes less time than seeing the GP in two or three separate visits. Plus, it means the GP is not as rushed.

Having a healthcare coach would be particularly helpful in these situations as they can assist the patient in establishing whether they are experiencing more than one issue. No one should expect a patient to know how different medical conditions interact.

Complex conditions can be a significant challenge and are commonly associated with multiple hospital visits and costly care requirements. Such conditions may include diabetes, asthma or a disability, which means that when an acute medical problem, such as a broken bone, occurs, the other condition will have an impact on healing.

Using a coach to resolve this issue by supporting a GP in caring for the patient would provide holistic care. If we are better able to support people during medical consultations and at home, everyone would benefit.

As mentioned before, doctors also have limited time to ensure that patients understand their diagnosis. If a doctor spends time to describe the condition and answer questions, and then is seen again once a patient has had time to think about what has been said, it is costly.

Instead, doctors could be supported by a healthcare coach to ensure that the patient and their family understand the doctor's diagnosis and the treatment they prescribe. This would provide patients and their families with adequate time to understand what is happening, and would be an inexpensive option that significantly improves the patient experience.

Part-time GPs and our transitional lifestyles affect our developing a relationship with our local GP.

There is one other consideration that needs addressing: GPs are increasingly working part-time. They also take holidays, like everyone else, which means they may not always be available when you need them. But if you see the same GP regularly, they will often have a colleague who they discuss patients with. They will typically recommend this person as a point of contact when they are away.

If you have not seen your GP for a while, then they may not let you know when they will be on holidays, but the receptionist will be able to direct you. This is also relevant if you need to see a GP quickly and your usual doctor is away for a couple of days.

Large clinics, sometimes called 'super care' or 'bulk-billing clinics', are becoming more common to provide better patient coverage where individual GPs are working fewer hours. These clinics are often open for long hours and have a team of GPs who work together to provide coverage. Again, I reiterate, it is always best to find a GP you trust.

If you choose this type of clinic, you have every right to request a particular GP. Ask the receptionist for the next time that the GP is available or scheduled to work so that you can attend the clinic at that time. Typically, these clinics won't make appointments, but when you arrive you can request to see the GP who is your preferred practitioner. It is your healthcare and requesting a specific GP is well within your rights.

Despite the various ways medical practices are evolving to better serve the patient, Medicare-funded allied healthcare plans cannot currently cover coaches. There is no support in our existing government funding for an experienced coach to help people through the health, welfare, disability or aged service industry.

The concept of a healthcare coach needs to be taken into consideration when the government attempts to develop projects that redirect patients to a GP. Patients will continue to go to the emergency department since it still costs nothing and they can have testing performed immediately and onsite. Effective programs should factor this in by having GP clinics co-located with pathology and radiology laboratories so that patients can receive testing results and medical care more quickly.

Chapter Three

The Promise of Public Health

According to the CDC Foundation, public health is 'the science of protecting and improving the health of people and their communities. This work is achieved by promoting healthy lifestyles, researching disease and injury prevention, and detecting, preventing and responding to infectious diseases.'[3]

While this definition is universal, the public health services that support its delivery have significant differences globally. In Australia, these services are largely funded through Medicare, whereas private health services are funded through insurance that an individual has chosen to contribute to.

The first few months for a parent of a newborn are filled with regular visits to the local Maternal and Child Health Centre. The Maternal Health nurse checks the baby's weight, various patterns of behaviour, and its movement, making sure that it's developing as expected.

Throughout primary and secondary education, schools send letters home to notify parents of a visit from the community nurse. Medical research has

---

3   'What is Public Health?' CDC Foundation. Accessed February 11, 2022. cdcfoundation.org/what-public-health.

shown that vaccinating children can help prevent a range of diseases. To effectively administer this vaccination program, governments partner with local schools to immunise children of the appropriate age.

When the child reaches their teenage years and enters secondary school, parents may also be advised of free access to dental health.

Many parents and children take this journey as a given. But without necessarily realising it, both are taking part in numerous examples of public health.

At all levels of government, public health policy is important. It is society's organised response to protect and promote health and prevent illness, injury and disability. It allows children to grow, develop and learn on the path to higher levels of education, leading to various forms of employment or the creation of businesses.

Prior to 2020, less than 2% of Australia's national health expenditure was on public health programs, yet the return far outweighed the cost.

During the past twenty to thirty years, the most significant public health programs have included:

1. *A reduction in neural tube defects in newborns.* Neural tube defects are severe birth deformities with a high mortality rate. Those babies that do survive persist with a lifelong disability. The 1990s saw the development of health promotion programs to encourage increased folate intake for women before and during pregnancy. This has reduced the risk of neural tube defects by up to

70%. The current recommendation is for a dietary supplement of folic acid under the guidance of the treating clinician.

2. *The National Immunisation Program.* As a partnership between federal, state and territory governments, free vaccines for eighteen diseases are available to all eligible people.[4] Immunisations have been shown to be very effective in decreasing the number of people affected by the diseased they've been vaccinated against.

3. *The National Cervical Screening Program.* This program promotes a human papillomavirus (HPV) cervical screening test every five years for women aged between 25 and 74.[5] Research shows that HPV is responsible for nearly all cases of cervical cancer. Hence this screening test replaced the old Pap test, which has more than halved the prevalence of cervical cancer in women since 1982. Researchers expect that if current vaccination and screening rates are maintained, cervical cancer is likely to be eliminated as a public health issue in Australia by 2035.[6]

---

4   'National Immunisation Program Schedule', Department of Health and Aged Care. Accessed July 12, 2022. health.gov.au/health-topics/immunisation/when-to-get-vaccinated/national-immunisation-program-schedule.

5   'National Cervical Screening Program', Department of Health and Aged Care. Accessed July 12, 2022. health.gov.au/initiatives-and-programs/national-cervical-screening-program.

6   'Eliminating cervical cancer in Australia by 2035', Cancer Council NSW. Accessed July 12, 2022. cancercouncil.com.au/research-pt/eliminating-cervical-cancer-in-australia-by-2035.

4. *Dental decay prevention.* The community water fluoridation program first began in the 1960s, but involvement varied across the country. Nowadays, fluoridated water is available to 89% of Australians. Lifelong access to fluoridated water has dramatically reduced tooth decay in adults. Other factors that impact oral health include the consumption of sugar, tobacco and alcohol, the practice of good oral hygiene and access to regular dental check-ups. Unfortunately, Medicare largely excludes the funding of public dental services. To combat this, the Medicare Teen Dental Plan was introduced in 2008, which then became the Child Dental Benefits Schedule in 2014. This program enables access to dental services, including examinations, x-rays, cleanings, fillings, root canals and extractions. However, it remains underutilised, as only 30% of eligible children use it.

5. *A reduction of skin cancers.* Slip! Slop! Slap! was launched by the Cancer Council in 1981 and is one of Australia's greatest success stories in the prevention of skin cancers. Due to its geographical positioning, Australia experiences great weather. But before the 1980s, most Australians were not mindful of sun damage and now Australia has one of the highest rates of skin cancer in the world in people over the age of forty. The original

Slip! Slop! Slap! campaign evolved into the SunSmart campaign, extending into schools, workplaces, the Surf Life Saving community, and the fashion, television and movie industries. This campaign has succeeded due to its integration across the community, government and workplace and because of the support of all political parties. The Slip! Slop! Slap! slogan was extended in 2008 to include 'Seek and Slide'. This refers seeking shade and sliding on sunglasses, all in an effort to avoid harmful effects from the sun. The SunSmart program is supported by the Centre for Behavioural Research in Cancer. This research is internationally recognized and seeks to identify the most effective ways to change behaviour that increases cancer risk.[7]

6. *A reduction in the number of deaths due to smoking.* Smoking has been shown to lead to one of the worst negative health outcomes that humanity has inflicted on itself. It remains the leading preventable cause of death and disease in Australia, contributing to many types of cancer, heart disease, stroke, stomach ulcers, and chest and lung diseases. Programs within Australia began with television ads showing the impact of smoking

---

7   'SunSmart Program', SunSmart. Accessed July 12, 2022. sunsmart. com.au/about-sunsmart/sunsmart-program.

on health. This extended to warnings on cigarette packaging and now includes Quit-line, an assistance service helping people overcome addiction to tobacco. Daily smoking rates for Australians aged 18 and older have dropped from 20% in 2001 to 12% in 2019, and there are now more people who have quit smoking at some point in their lives than people who currently smoke.[8]

7. *National Road Safety Strategy.* First established in 1992,[9] this ten-year plan focused on developing a framework for national road safety. It includes many elements—road and roadside infrastructure, vehicle safety, lower speed limits (for example, in school zones), and behavioural programs covering drink driving, seat belts and speed. Trauma and death associated with road accidents, while reduced significantly since this program began, remain a big issue for the community. The National Road Safety Strategy 2021–2030 targets a further 50% reduction in the annual number of fatalities and a 30% reduction in the annual number of serious injuries. This is to be achieved through safe roads, improved public transport, safe vehicles, and safe road use, with

---

8   'Smoking Statistic', Better Health Channel. Accessed July 12, 2022. better-health.vic.gov.au/health/healthyliving/smoking-statistics.

9   'National Road Saftey Strategy 2011–2020', Australian Transportation Council. Accessed July 9, 2022. roadsafety.gov.au/sites/default/files/2019-11/nrss_2011_2020.pdf.

speed management a key element in each of the areas.[10]

8. *A reduction in gun deaths.* Following the Port Arthur Massacre in 1996, where thirty-five people were killed and twenty-three injured, the Howard Government introduced the National Firearms Agreement. This included a buy-back provision, and the ownership of automatic and semi-automatic weapons became limited to licensed individuals who used firearms for more than just their personal protection. The agreement continues to have support from all levels of government, and there have been no public mass shootings since that time. With the reduction in gun ownership there has also been a drop in the rate of firearm and homicide suicide.[11]

9. *A low prevalence of HIV and AIDS.* From the outset, the response to the AIDS epidemic within Australia was led by the community. Leaders called for a strong awareness and increased research to understand the magnitude of the problem. Peer-led prevention and support brought together many volunteers, political leaders, governments,

10   'National Road Saftey Strategy 2021–30', Australian Transportation Council. Accessed July 9, 2022. roadsafety.gov.au/sites/default/files/documents/National-Road-Safety-Strategy-2021-30.pdf.

11   Ramchand, Rajeev and Jessica Saunders, 'The Effects of the 1996 National Firearms Agreement in Australia on Suicide, Homicide and Mass Shootings.' Rand Corporation. Accessed July 9, 2022. rand.org/research/gun-policy/analysis/essays/1996-national-firearms-agreement.html.

affected communities, those living with HIV, researchers and the health profession.[12] For many years since then, Australia has focused on safe sex and needle and syringe exchange programs within key communities.

10. *Preventing deaths from bowel and breast cancer.* BreastScreen Australia programs grant women over 40 a free mammography every two years. By detecting the disease early, the program aims to reduce illness and death. Advances in screening and treatment have seen a fall of 35% in age-standardised breast cancer deaths for women. Women who are diagnosed now have a 92% chance of surviving for five years.[13] Meanwhile, the National Bowel Cancer Screening Program was established in 2006, which saw the first introduction of a program for bowel cancer testing. This program was later improved by expanding the initial target age range to include more people. Eligible Australians between the ages of 50 and 74 are sent a free, simple test that can be done in the home.[14] Bowel cancer can develop without any symptoms and can grow undetected

12   'Our History', Australian Federation of AIDS Organizations. Accessed July 9, 2022. afao.org.au/about-afao/history/.

13   'Breast Cancer in Australia Statistics', Cancer Australia. Accessed July 12, 2022. canceraustralia.gov.au/cancer-types/breast-cancer/statistics.

14   'National Bowel Cancer Screening Program', Department of Health and Aged Care. Accessed July 12, 2022. health.gov.au/initiatives-and-programs/national-bowel-cancer-screening-program.

before spreading to other parts of the body. For this reason, having a screening process is very important. It is estimated that early detection of bowel cancer will save some 35,000 lives over the course of thirty years.[15]

Australians have benefited from a world-class health system that has allowed them to live long, healthy lives and travel the globe. Maladies that were once feared, such as polio, have become distant memories or been entirely forgotten.

The safety net provided by vaccines is intangible, but very real, as the COVID pandemic has reminded us.

---

15   'Top 10 Public Health Successes Over the Last 20 Years,' Public Health Association Australia, accessed 11 February 2022, phaa.net.au/documents/item/3241.

Chapter Four

The COVID-19 Pandemic

The effectiveness of the National Immunisation Program in Australia has seen a very low incidence of vaccine-preventable diseases. Its success has come from funding by state, territory and Australian governments, delivery through maternal child centres and schools, and availability to other relevant age and risk groups, free of charge.

With many diseases rarely visible, it has been easy for the community and healthcare providers to become complacent and lose sight of how protected they were.

All these factors came into the public spotlight when we found ourselves in the midst of a crisis due to a global pandemic and the safe-guarding of public health became paramount.

It began in late December 2019, when Chinese authorities announced they were investigating a series of viral pneumonia cases with an unknown cause. Early January 2020 saw the Huanan Seafood Wholesale Market closed in Wuhan, where many people believe the disease originated. By 7 January 2020, Chinese authorities confirmed they had identified a novel coronavirus, Severe Acute Respiratory Syndrome Coronavirus 2 (SARS-CoV-2), as responsible for the disease. This virus became known as COVID-19.

As January progressed, cases began appearing outside of China. Very quickly, they skyrocketed, and associated deaths started being reported. Later that month, Australia confirmed its initial case of COVID-19. This was the first time in many years that the Australian community felt vulnerable to an unknown virus. On 30 January 2020, the World Health Organization (WHO) declared a global health emergency. The Australian Prime Minister, Scott Morrison, then activated an emergency response plan on 27 February 2020. A few weeks later, on 11 March 2020, the WHO declared COVID-19 a global pandemic.

As the number of cases increased around the globe, the Australian government closed its borders to all nonresidents on 20 March 2020, and all returning residents were required to quarantine for two weeks. Varying measures were implemented within Australia, with some states closing borders and introducing social distancing restrictions. These decisions were made to sustain the delivery of healthcare to those who would potentially need it most and to prevent the system from becoming overwhelmed.

In Victoria, following a breach of protocol at a designated quarantine hotel, case numbers surged through May and June. This prompted a strict lockdown that ultimately lasted four months. People were only allowed to leave home for essential work and supplies or for exercise, and could only travel within a 5 km radius of their home.

These measures interrupted various aspects of normal life: travel, work, school, entertainment, sporting events, concerts and festivals. Many activities were cancelled, working from home became common, and schools had to transition rapidly to online learning. The social and economic impacts were severe.

The restrictions due to the second wave of cases finally ended in Victoria on 28 October 2020, after 112 days.

Over the ensuing months, there were various outbreaks in different states, resulting in borders closing and some restrictions being reimposed, then relaxed as case numbers declined.

With Pfizer and Astra-Zeneca vaccines approved, the national vaccination program began on 22 February 2021. Soon after, in April 2021, a quarantine-free travel bubble opened between Australia and New Zealand. It was the first glimpse of a return to normality.

However, the sense that the pandemic was abating was short-lived. In late May 2021, Victoria entered another lockdown as a cluster of cases increased. Testing revealed the prevalence of a new variant, known as Delta. Restrictions became a rollercoaster, increasing as case numbers went up and then being withdrawn as case numbers declined. Gradually, the Delta variant became more widespread, extending across other states. The travel bubble with New Zealand was suspended, and borders closed once again.

This variant had a shorter incubation time, was highly transmissible, and had a higher severity of symptoms. Mechanisms that were effective in the first twelve months, such as contact tracing, struggled with the overload of increasing numbers.

The strategy shifted to getting people immunised as quickly as possible. With the increased availability of vaccines, eligibility was expanded from aged people and frontline workers to the broader community over the age of 18. Children under that age were also later approved for vaccination.

Case numbers increased from late June 2021, peaking between late September and mid-October. In mid-December 2021, the numbers began to increase again.[16] This time, it was the emergence of another variant known as Omicron. This variant appeared to be less severe, but highly transmissible, overtaking the rate of any previous variants. Case numbers skyrocketed again, and there was an increase in associated hospital admissions. The demand for services meant that category 2 and 3 elective surgeries were suspended to allow the system to cope.

The introduction of Rapid Antigen Tests (RATs) enabled individuals to check if they were positive without having to queue at a Polymerase Chain Reaction (PCR) testing site. This was helpful within the community, as pathology laboratories were not

16   'Coronavirus (COVID-19) at a glance – 31 December 2021', Department of Health and Aged Care. Accessed July 12, 2022. health.gov.au/resources/publications/coronavirus-covid-19-at-a-glance-31-december-2021.

keeping up with the demand and results were taking days instead of hours to be returned.

As February 2022 drew to a close, school students returned to the classroom without a dramatic increase in cases, workers returned to offices, and the requirements for mask wearing were relaxed. Health authorities, in conjunction with government leaders, focused on continuing to moving forward in a manner that allows the economy to recover without unduly inundating the health system.

Throughout the pandemic, the response shifted according to the level of knowledge about the virus. Extreme outbreaks were contained through systems of contact tracing, which allowed authorities to identify close connections of those infected and test them quickly. Isolation was enforced for the person returning a positive result and their close contacts.

Investing in public health measures is good for everyone. While some restrictions have been challenging during the pandemic, Australia has so far been able to minimise COVID's impact on its populace. The case-fatality ratio stood at 0.2%, or 4,966 deaths, as of 23 February 2022, which is on a par with other countries that have been able to keep their cases contained. The differences between countries for the number of cases and deaths can be attributed to accessibility to testing, the capacity of the health infrastructure, and demographics of the population.

The pandemic led to the compulsory wearing of masks, social distancing, the shuttering of nonessential businesses, restricted travel, and the closure of state borders. These measures minimised the demand for hospitals, which ensured an adequate capacity to treat those who became seriously ill.

The public health response, however, came with an associated economic cost, and the fiscal years 2019–20 and 2020–21 have seen an unprecedented level of government expenditure to support those financially who are affected. Some of the expenses have included:

- $89bn through the jobkeeper program, which provided wage support for 3.8 million Australians
- $35bn in cashflow payments supporting 800,000 businesses and not-for-profit organisations
- $20bn supplement payment made to 3 million Australians participating in the jobseeker program

These are just a few of the measures the Australian government committed to in the 2021 federal budget. In all, there was a total of $311bn allocated to fight COVID-19.[17]

Seeing travel opportunities and normal day-to-day movement suddenly curtailed because of COVID-19 was confronting. In a world of consumerism, where products and services are often created before there

---

17 'The 2021 federal budget reveals huge $311bn cost of Covid to Australian economy', The Guardian. Accessed July 12, 2022. theguardian.com/australia-news/2021/may/11/federal-budget-2021-papers-reveals-huge-cost-of-covid-australian-government-economy-economic-stimulus-packages.

is a need for them, there was a sense of vulnerability when a solution was not immediately available.

Vaccine development is complicated and lengthy. They cannot be developed at the speed the public has come to expect from other products and services. There is intense rigour, and the standards used for measuring progress often make it slow, ensuring each stage is successful before moving to the next.

The Therapeutic Goods Administration (TGA) in Australia regulates medications through premarket assessment. They license Australian manufacturers and verify the compliance of those overseas, making sure they meet the same standards as their domestic counterparts. Once medications are brought to market, the TGA continues to monitor and ensure standards are enforced.

The speed with which vaccines were approved and made available locally was a testament to the cooperation of international scientific communities, and the collaboration of global manufacturing and distribution.

During the pandemic, the government has required robust scientific data and analysis before considering a vaccine candidate. They have contributed significant funds in research and development to assist the global effort in developing a vaccine as quickly as possible.

Vaccines are an important factor in the economic recovery of the broader Pacific and South East Asia region. They also reduce the burden of COVID-19 and assist in opening up the region for travel and the transfer of goods. To this end, Australia has committed $623.2 million to assist countries within this region with access to vaccines.[18]

The vaccination program began in February 2021, focusing on those people who were at higher risk of serious illness were they to contract COVID-19 and those most likely to be exposed to it—quarantine and border workers, frontline healthcare workers, and aged care and disability care workers and residents. Elderly adults over 70 years of age were also included.

The next phase focused on adults aged over 50 and Aboriginal and Torres Strait Islander people. The following phase included the remaining adult population. With the prevalence of the Delta and Omicron variants, vaccines have been made available to children as well.

As of 11 July, 2022, over 95% of people aged 16 and over are fully vaccinated. This rate, however, is not consistent across all communities. As of 5 July 2022, some Aboriginal and Torres Strait Islander groups have vaccination rates as low as 65.1%, with the highest vaccination rate being 89.5%.[19]

In Australia, the most vulnerable communities are often the most remote. They may be located hundreds of kilometres from larger, established towns and cities. Aboriginal and Torres Strait Islander communities are the first inhabitants of this country—herewith referred to as First Nations communities. They have

---

18   See note 4 above.

19   'COVID-19 Vaccination Roll-out', Operation COVID Shield. Accessed July 12, 2022. health.gov.au/sites/default/files/documents/2022/07/covid-19-vaccine-rollout-update-12-july-2022.pdf.

a range of existing health and socioeconomic inequities that increase their vulnerability to COVID-19. They also have a higher percentage of underlying chronic conditions. When Delta became the dominant strain, the First Nations communities were disproportionately affected. The ongoing challenge is to work with the communities and leaders to deepen the understanding of the importance of vaccination and COVID-safe practices.

At the best of times, administering public health across diverse communities is a complex process. This complexity is exacerbated when significant economic factors are involved. The appropriate balance can only come through some level of trial and error, research and a willingness to collaborate across all levels of government, business and the community. Despite the high level of vaccination, there are concerns associated with the vaccines. How long will they last? How effective will they be against new strains of the virus? A booster was recommended in response to Omicron. What might the side effects be in the long term?

Given that vaccines normally take ten years to develop, these concerns are to be expected. The public wants to trust that the vaccines are safe and effective. With this in mind, their development process needs to be transparent. Ongoing studies must measure the vaccines' effectiveness and discover any potential long-term side effects.

COVID-19 is here to stay in some form. Living with it effectively will be the challenge.

Chapter Five

Cracks in the Healthcare System

Australia's healthcare system works in silos or specialities that limit the context of a person's care. Medical staff grow proficient in the treatment and care of specific illnesses, while learning very little about others outside their area of expertise.

If a patient contacts the healthcare system with a traumatic injury to their hand, a surgical hand specialist is required and a physiotherapist will help them through rehabilitation. But unless the patient is asked, no one discusses the ongoing impact of the injury for the patient. They may have worked in an environment that requires hand dexterity. They may be the main breadwinner. They may have a child at home with a hearing disability and need to be able to use their hand to talk with their child.

This is just one example of how a seemingly simple thing can have an ongoing impact on the life of a patient.

Research into healthcare has also become specialised. Treatments have improved as a result and hospitals have become centres of healthcare excellence. Nowadays, Australia is regarded as world-class when it comes to medical research.

Medicine is ideally premised on evidence-based practice, which is when the healthcare professional bases their diagnosis and treatment on the most current research. In most cases, this is appropriate, but occasionally people do not fit the current evidence. This most often occurs with women or people with multiple medical conditions.

Most medical research uses healthy, wealthy, white men in their twenties. This obscures the effects of interactions between medical conditions. Unfortunately, this means that ordinary people may not fit nicely into the evidence. Healthcare professionals need to consider when it is important to use evidence-based practice and when this strategy may not work.

Given that medical research improves our understanding of certain conditions, it does enable us to provide guidelines on how to best treat a patient's medical condition.

We have made some extraordinary medical breakthroughs in the last century that have had an astounding impact on the lifestyles of everyday people. Children and mothers are less likely to die during childbirth. Children are also less likely to have typical childhood infections that only a century ago would have been deadly or caused lifelong disability. Most babies born today in Australia are likely to live long, healthy lives, so we have smaller families and are now able to provide them with good food and education.

Medicine has almost done *too* well. Now people are questioning why medicine provides the care it does. Vaccinations are a good example of this. We no longer see the effects of serious infectious diseases, such as polio or measles. We really do not know how lucky we are.

But medicine sometimes makes mistakes as well. People have been given drugs for one condition that have in turn caused a different one. The research was not exhaustive enough, and there were serious side effects that occurred when patients started using the drug that only appeared after they were on the medication for a longer time than the studies lasted.

Only two decades ago, we had a new wonder drug that could help people with inflammation. Earlier treatments had the side effect of inducing stomach ulcers, and people who were on the earlier medication had to be put on a second medication to counteract this risk. The new drug treatment became a regular script and was widely used for people with arthritis. After five years, it became evident that increased numbers of people were having strokes and heart attacks after taking this drug for a long time. As soon as these side effects became known the drug was recalled, but some people had already died or had become permanently disabled.

Medicine is learning to be more conservative, but large research and development firms exist to make money. It is a highly regulated system in Australia, but it still makes mistakes.

**Ten years of misdiagnoses led Rayna
to have an impaired immune system.**

In 1988, a young traveller, Rayna, returned from the tropics with chronic vomiting and diarrhoea. She was able to hold down some food and drink, but the condition was pretty constant. She was at university and had trouble completing her degree. She was often unwell and had sporadic stomach pains. She went from being extraordinarily fit to being constantly unwell. Being young, she continued to travel and did not stay in one place very long. When her condition worsened, she would see a new GP. But the treatment she was provided did not last.

Sometimes, the GP would give her antibiotics. Other times, the GP would give her medication to treat stomach ulcers. Occasionally, if she saw the same GP over a few visits, she was sent to see a gastroenterologist who specialised in stomach pain, diarrhoea and vomiting. The gastroenterologist would perform surgery and then provide her with antibiotics and medication for stomach ulcers.

If she went back to the same GP, he would then refer her for psychological assessment by either a psychiatrist or a psychologist. They assessed her for anorexia or bulimia. She was given a clean bill of health, but then she moved and the cycle would repeat. At every appointment, she told the doctor or specialist that the condition started during her travels through the tropics.

Her family and friends thought she was 'putting it on' and worried that she was anorexic. This caused problems with her relationships because people were tired of hearing about it. She struggled to finish university and her work life suffered. Finally, in 1998—ten years later—a good friend suggested she see an infectious disease specialist. Her friend was a nurse and had discussed her situation with one of her medical colleagues, who gave her the name of a particular specialist. Rayna made the appointment, but she felt downhearted. She had begun to think that maybe her body was just built that way.

Rayna went to the appointment and told her story again; that it started while she was travelling in the tropics; that she had ongoing stomach pain, diarrhoea and vomiting; and that her weight was the same as she was when she was sixteen.

The specialist listened to her story. The assessment lasted an hour. At the end of it, he said, 'You are likely to have one of five conditions. Luckily for you, the treatment for every one of those conditions is the same.' He asked her to take some further tests but gave her the right antibiotic for her condition. She had to take the antibiotic for two weeks.

Rayna was finally cured after ten years and two weeks. On the downside, she finally started putting on weight and had to watch what she ate for the first time. Unfortunately, Rayna's immune system had been damaged due to the many years of infection.

Karen's misdiagnosis led to inappropriate treatments and conflict in her family.

One day in 2002, a new mother, Karen, awoke and found she could not move; her joints were too stiff. After a while, she managed to get herself up using simple over-the-counter pain relief. She was a young mother and had to care for her new baby.

She called her mother for help and went to see her local GP. He thought from her description that she had signs of rheumatoid arthritis. She was sent to a specialist, who after hearing her story, came to the same conclusion. But before starting Karen on medications, the specialist felt she needed to do some tests. The tests came back clear, to everyone's surprise, so Karen was told it was probably osteoarthritis and put on opiates to manage the pain.

After five years of trying different pain medications, she ended up seeing another rheumatologist. This rheumatologist received the same results from the same tests, but she remained unconvinced—so she ordered another test. This was not a standard test, so it cost Karen a bit to have it done. But she really wanted to stop relying on opiates to manage her pain, so she paid to have it done. This new test showed that Karen had rheumatoid arthritis throughout her body, not osteoarthritis as it was earlier presumed.

Some tests are not 100% reliable, but the first tests she received were considered to be highly reliable for the condition. Unfortunately, she was one of the few people who do not have the result one would expect.

For five years, then, Karen was on a variety of pain medications, but none of them were the right medication. Because her pain appeared to have no identifiable reason, Karen was repeatedly sent to psychologists to see if she had a psychological reason for her pain levels. Each time, Karen was cleared by the psychologist. But it was a difficult time because she was trying to manage a young baby. She was unable to return to work, which put pressure on her marriage. Once her pain was better controlled, her home life went back to normal, she was able to care well for her baby, and eventually Karen went back to work.

Sometimes, people with a diagnosis are given information about their illness and treatment, but not about how this condition may affect their everyday life.

There are also times when people have developed a condition that medicine does not understand and they are sent away without it being treated, or they are sent to different specialists with no actual outcome. As a result, they become disillusioned and may end up losing their ability to continue working, or family and friends may think they are 'putting on' their symptoms to get attention.

They may also require ongoing treatment to prevent the condition from worsening, though they may not realise it. Preventative treatments are often not continued by the patient due to confusion about their effectiveness.

Finally, if their medical condition is chronic (long-term), they may not get referred to community services that can help them. Often, this is because doctors may not know what services exist to help their patients in the community.

But medical diagnosis and treatment are not the only specialised forms of healthcare in Australia.

Chapter Six

The Dental Care Element

Another readily recognisable silo of healthcare is dental care. In Australia, dentistry is largely a competitive, private industry. If an individual requires dental care and they do not have private healthcare or cannot afford a private appointment, there is a long wait for public care. Sometimes, it can take months or even years.

Due to an amendment to the constitution,[20] the Australian government cannot directly conscript any aspect of dental care (as with medical doctors—after all, dentists are doctors too). Therefore, dentists cannot be forced into working for the government.

Medicare does not subsidise dental services like it does medical care. State and territory governments provide public dental care but it is inadequate to cover the majority of people who require subsidised care.

Dentistry is largely under free-market control—that is, patients are expected to pay for most dental treatments independently. But there are not enough dentists, so this leads to competition in the market-

---

20   Section 51 xxiiiA of the Australian Constitution.

place in the larger towns and cities (not so in regional or remote areas).

Of course, this assumes that people can pay for dental care and can make a decision about that care in a competitive market—that is, that people have the time and circumstances to look around and find a dentist who has competitive rates and does good work.

Unfortunately, this is not what typically happens. People who are looking for a dentist are usually in a rush, dealing with their everyday lives. They typically go to a dentist near home. Once they find one who offers a suitable appointment, they often stay with them. Few people have the time and wherewithal to study the market.

Also, there are a few public dentistry centres that are available to treat those who cannot afford private dental care. These are typically available in large cities around Australia.

The federal government expects the states and territories to pay for public dental care. There are provisions in private health insurance that cover some of the costs of dental services, but these are limited. The cost for private dental care has become out of reach for most people in recent years as the cost of living has risen while wages have stagnated.

There are some community health services that provide publicly funded dental care. (For example, in most states and territories, there are school dental vans that provide assessment and advice to school children.) The waiting list for public dental services is almost always long (it can take years) unless you have an emergency (which even then can take several weeks). This means that many people do not have any form of dental care. The impact on the health of our Australian community is deeply concerning.

**The effect of not going to a dentist regularly
has had a large health impact on Max and,
as a consequence, on the Australian taxpayer.**

Max was a labourer who worked in a city that had reasonable working conditions and pretty regular work. He did well, but because of his irregular work, he moved around a bit. Still, he stayed in the same city and his family was nearby.

One day, he was working at a job and accidentally cut his hand. He went to the local emergency department and they put in five stitches. He was told to take a few days off work and given advice on how to treat his wound. He was told it should heal but he needed to see his GP to have the stitches removed in ten days.

He had just started his current job and was required to move from his old unit to one closer to the job, as the travel times were too long to manage.

This new job was going to be more stable and it was something he was good at, so he was quite pleased to have it. But he was on a contract so if he did not work, he did not get paid. Five days off was not too bad, though, since he could make it up.

After a few days, he felt like he had the flu. He started getting fevers and felt weak and a bit nauseated. He took himself down to see the GP. After a wait of four hours, he was finally called in.

He described his symptoms to the doctor, but the doctor was too busy looking at his computer and barely looked at Max during the appointment. The GP wrote a prescription for an antibiotic because of Max's fevers, and said to come back if the antibiotic did not work.

Two days later, Max called his sister Casey to take him back to the GP. Casey had two children, so she could not take him until the next day.

When Max went back to the GP clinic, he saw a different GP. This doctor was older and took his time. He looked at Max and asked him about the wound on his hand. Max said he had cut it at work and showed him the stitches. The GP assessed the hand and asked Max how he cut it. Max said he was working on some fencing at his new job, lost his concentration and accidentally cut his hand.

The GP looked at Max again and asked him if he had a sore throat. Max replied he did not have a sore throat, but his jaw was sore. The GP looked into Max's mouth and saw that he had some very serious-looking swelling around his upper teeth. There were some areas of black skin, which was not reassuring.

The GP asked Max if he had a dentist. He did not. He had not seen a dentist since he was a kid in school. The GP referred Max to the emergency department at the city's public dental hospital. Casey drove Max into the hospital but had to leave him to pick up the kids.

After a few hours, Max was seen by a dentist. He required the immediate removal of three teeth and his blood was taken to see if he had septicaemia. The dentist also asked Max about his diet, which was largely soft because chewing anything was painful.

Max had broken a tooth during a wrestle with his nephew several weeks earlier. He just left it because he could not afford to go to the dentist, and he was not aware that there was a public dentist he could have seen. His jaw had started becoming painful two weeks later, but he did not realise it had anything to do with his tooth.

The dentist organised for Max to be referred to a public hospital for treatment. The septicaemia was confirmed, and Max was also diagnosed with diabetes. He ended up needing surgery to have his jaw cleaned, as well as needing further stitches. He was in hospital for nearly two weeks so his septicaemia could be managed and the staff could educate him about his diabetes. His hand wound healed once he was on the right antibiotic, and he was discharged into community care.

In the meantime, Max's job had been given away and he could no longer pay the rent for his new unit, so he moved in with his sister. He had a lot of trouble finding new work after that.

He has now started a new apprenticeship, and he understands he can get regular dental checks through the local community health service. He is also getting diabetes care through the same community health service and his local GP.

As discussed earlier, dental care in Australia is largely funded through the private system. This means that many people do not attend to their teeth early enough for preventative treatment.

In Max's case, a visit to the dentist would have meant a clean and a filling where the tooth had broken. Instead, the taxpayer had to pay for three GP visits, a trip to emergency, surgery and two weeks in hospital. The diabetes may not have been picked up until later, but if the septicaemia had not been diagnosed, Max could have ended up even more unwell. In fact, he could have died. The complication of diabetes could have made this scenario even more serious.

Australians have been lucky in that most dental care is about prevention and, for those who can afford it, cosmetic treatment. If we consider that good dental health affects what we eat, and therefore our nutrition, and that infected teeth can have a very serious impact on our health, dental care is paramount. Cosmetic dental care can even be important for people's ability to socialise and to find and keep work. Missing front teeth can lead to people being judged negatively or isolating themselves socially.

For these reasons, dentistry needs to be added to the Medicare Benefits Scheme. Caring for our teeth is not just a cosmetic issue. It can have an effect on nutrition, social isolation related to the ability to eat as everyone else does, and the more serious issue of infection. Caring for our community requires that we make caring for teeth as important as any other medical need.

Chapter Seven

Aged Care and Its Options

With our ageing population, aged care has become an increasingly complex and confusing silo of healthcare. There are multiple programs and services to support chronically ill or disabled individuals and, as a result, people can be supported through many programs in their own home. This is the simplest level of aged care.

As someone's needs increase, they can go into supported accommodation for which there are multiple levels of care. One is minimal support, usually in a unit or apartment where there are others with similar needs. These complexes often support their community with hydrotherapy programs, a community hall with a library or cinema-style room, and excursions for shopping trips or other entertainment. This allows the facility's community to do things together, while also having their own space in their apartment or unit.

As a person's care needs increase, they move into what is commonly referred to as 'low-level care'. This is provided in a housing complex where each individual either has their own room or shares a room with another. A person requiring low-level care often needs help with things like showering, going to the toilet, eating meals, and moving around. The service provider may also provide a regular social program in the complex so that people can get out of their rooms and socialise.

'High-level care' (in comparison) is for individuals who require continuous medical support for their chronic illnesses, which may include things like special medications requiring constant monitoring, special feeding equipment, and chronic wound management. They may also be unable to walk and so need to be moved regularly in bed and have to be in a caring and supportive environment. These complexes often have highly-trained nursing staff working full-time.

The aged care system appears sensible, but again it is complex and confusing. The My Aged Care program commenced at a similar time as the NDIS. These federally funded programs are trying to provide independence and appropriate care for the individual. Instead of service providers being funded to provide the care, the individual is given funding to spend on what they believe will help them. The complex and confusing part is that each person is expected to know what level of care they require and how to access that care. Then, they're responsible for selecting their coverage from a large number of providers in a highly competitive market. So, it's hard to know which one is best for the individual's specific needs.

My Aged Care has a website that can help people navigate service provision, but this assumes that individuals have the capacity to navigate a website, read well, and understand what it is they need.

The current statistics on literacy indicate that this is not the case for many people. A large portion of the Australian community simply cannot read. Australia also has a diverse and complex multicultural population. Even if they can read and navigate the websites set up to help them, many people have little, if any, previous experience in healthcare.

Rose had a large family who were actively involved in her care.

Family was very important to them. However, their experience with the aged care system tore the family apart.

Anna's grandmother, Rose, was an active woman who travelled regularly for her passion, which was lawn bowls. She entered competitions and was regularly involved in a wide-ranging community.

She also had a large family. Rose had twelve children and over twenty grandchildren. Most of her children had completed university and were married, and two had passed away already.

On a routine trip to another state in Australia, she competed in a lawn bowls competition. During her holiday, she developed a headache, but with rest and some headache medication, she was fine. She had headaches on and off before the trip and had seen a GP about them, but he was not concerned.

Rose was considered a strong woman by her family. She had lived in relative poverty during the early years of her marriage because her husband Bob was disabled. He had contracted polio as a child and had medical problems throughout his life. Bob could only work sporadically. So, Rose had to manage the children and find ways to supplement their income.

They lived on a farm and tried to grow crops and had goats and chickens. Some days, she struggled to put together a meal. But she was hardworking and managed to support her children into university.

On the return trip from her travel interstate, her headache got worse. She started to show signs of confusion. Her lawn bowls team rushed her home. She went into hospital and then on to a rehabilitation hospital.

They could not find what was wrong, but the medical team thought she had had a stroke. Over the next few months, she deteriorated significantly and required a high level of care.

She could become aggressive at times, but her confusion was the most challenging part. The family found it confronting and upsetting. The strong woman they knew had become a completely different person, a shell of who she had been. Rose was still quite agile, but she could not shower herself or take herself to the toilet. If left alone, she would not eat.

The rehabilitation team met with her family and told them that Rose required constant care. They recommended putting her into an aged care facility.

Her son Cameron had a unit at the back of his three-bedroom, single-storey home. The family wanted to manage her at home, so the rehabilitation team provided education to the family on how to manage her care needs. They also provided the family with resources to find support, if needed. So, the family took her home and shared the care between them.

After several months, they realised it was too hard. Rose required 24-hour monitoring. She stayed up at night and if the family were not alert, she would escape the unit. The house was on a main road, so it was unsafe for her to be wandering alone.

The family had started to fight about things that happened and about who was caring for Rose and when. They tried getting some support at home, but it was too confusing and her care needs became increasingly hard to manage.

Eventually, Rose returned to the rehabilitation hospital. The hospital did another scan, which picked up just how significant the stroke was. After many meetings with the family, she was put into care.

The family was heartbroken, since they knew just how much their mother feared such places. To provide her with the best care possible, they sold the family farm. This gave them enough money to place her in their preferred aged care home. Rose was in care for many years, but it took the family many more years to stop fighting.

If the family had been supported better through the grieving stages of losing the person they thought of as their Mum and had been provided with timely information about homecare services to support them in caring for her needs at home, this may have helped them through the process of giving up her care.

If a healthcare coach was involved in the process, they would have met regularly with the family to see how things were going. When things started to become increasingly more difficult, they could have suggested relevant support services, like home help, Meals on Wheels, respite and counselling for the family, all while working alongside the GP to ensure the best care possible for Rose. The coach could have shown the family the My Aged Care website, so they could look through the services available and the different aged care homes nearby when the time came to put her into a care facility.

Sometimes, families can be more focused on what their mother or father wanted than on the reality of what that choice will mean to their lives. In an effort to abide by Rose's wishes, there may have been nothing the family would have done differently. But at least they would have felt heard and supported by the GP and his team.

Chapter Eight

The Growth of Disability Services

The disability sector is also experiencing unprecedented reforms with the introduction of the NDIS. This is driving an enormous change in the way disability services are provided and has brought people with a disability out from behind closed doors and into mainstream conversation. The effect of this has already been astounding. The disabled are being considered in many areas of public life like never before, and inclusive policy is becoming a mainstream topic in workplace culture.

Before the NDIS, disability services were largely managed by the state or territory governments. Australia has a disability pension so that people can live, but it was, and still is, insufficient to manage both the care needs of a person with a disability and their living expenses. The disability support pension is the living wage (for rent, utilities and food), and the NDIS provides funds for families who require extra support to help the person with a disability learn life skills, provide respite care for the main caregiver, or support the person with a disability to get work or to attend social activities.

At the same time, our social welfare system provides people who are out of work with a living wage to help them with food, clothes and shelter. It is inadequate and access is difficult.

These two systems do not interact except that people on a disability support pension may also qualify for the NDIS. (This is based on their assessed disability, not on the fact they have a pension.)

As a result, many disabled people live in poverty. Until recently, it was common for them to be handed over to the state or territory for management. This was heartbreaking, but few families could afford the cost of services and equipment.

Segregated schools were developed to support the educational needs of people with a disability, which aided a significant number of families and allowed them to have time to work or rest. But when a child finished school, there was little support available. Many families broke down under the pressure as the financial and physical stress became too much.

When people with a disability became adults, there were very few services available to provide them with meaningful work or lifestyle. They were often left at home, isolated. They might go to day centres that provided them with some sense of community, but the number of these was limited and had very long waiting lists. If the family could no longer care for them at home, they would often be placed in aged care homes or similar facilities. This gave the disabled little hope of a meaningful existence.

In addition, people with a mental health disability have been largely left out of appropriate services. Many of our Australian homeless community are people with mental health issues, often a psychiatric condition such as severe depression, bipolar disorder or schizophrenic disorders. Some turn to alcohol or drug abuse. This group of disabled people can also be found in our jail system because they have turned to crime. They are often the targets of abuse, as it is too easy for people to see them as 'not human'.

Given the above, the rollout of the NDIS is extraordinarily significant. It has enormously increased the funding available in the community to support the disabled. We need to make sure that families are better supported and able to work, and that people with a disability will be given purposeful assistance to have meaningful lives, whether through paid employment or engagement in social activities.

One family's journey through the disability services.

Ava's disability caused severe family trauma, but they are now better supported and remain together.

Michelle was a nurse and a new mother. Her daughter, Ava, was a happy baby who brought Michelle and her husband enormous joy. Brian and Michelle had met later in life, and when Ava was born, they were really excited.

When Ava turned twenty months, however, she became withdrawn and would not answer to her name. At first, Michelle and Brian thought there might be something wrong with her hearing, so little Ava had surgery.

The specialist thought that Ava would hear again and she would be back to her old self in a week. A week passed, and another, and another. Ava's behaviour did not improve.

So, they went to another specialist, a developmental paediatrician. This doctor could see from the first meeting that Ava had classic symptoms of autism. It was unusual to see a female at this level of the spectrum. He recommended they start Ava on an intensive therapy program to help her reconnect with the world.

Michelle and Brian had saved quite a bit during their early years, so they paid for the therapy. There were no government supports at the time, so it was very expensive. Ava went on a waiting list for government assistance, but it would be three years before that commenced. By then, Ava was at school.

The extensive therapy program did help Ava. She was able to pay attention to her education and she was her happy self again. When the government supports started, they were not much.

Because of the cost for therapy and the time it required, Michelle and Brian had used all their saved money, and Michelle was not able to go back to work. The financial strain was too much, and Michelle and Brian were struggling. Their relationship took second place to Ava's needs.

But soon after, Ava started going to a special school and made it very clear she no longer wanted to continue therapy. She still could not speak, but her communication was very clear. She would get very distressed when the therapists arrived at their home.

Michelle and Brian decided to not continue with the therapy. They took respite where they could with the small amount of government assistance they received, but they could no longer afford the extra support and Ava's needs remained quite high.

Michelle was physically fatigued and started getting sick a lot. Brian was struggling to manage work and whatever needed to be done around the house. He became distressed that he could not manage to make ends meet. He took pride in his work and had achieved a lot, but it was not enough.

Then, early in Ava's second year of school, things took a turn for the worse. Ava was playing with Michelle late one evening and she accidentally hit her mother in the face. The blow was quite hard, and Michelle ended up losing her sight. Having two disabled people in the home was very difficult.

Finally, after two years, the NDIS started in their area. For the first time in six years,

Michelle and Brian were getting the support they needed.

Brian was able to go to work without worrying about what would happen if he was not home. He was able to catch up on those things at home that needed fixing, much to his relief.

Brian and Michelle were able to manage to go out as a couple for the first time in a long while. Michelle's rehabilitation was stable, and she learned new skills that allowed her to find work again. Things were much better for everyone.

The NDIS is still being rolled out, so there are still communities that have not received this level of support yet. The change is significant whenever the NDIS moves into an area, and everyone is finding it to be a challenge. Families are unsure what supports to ask for and service providers are strained due to the difference in how they are funded.

There is a lot of media coverage as well, both positive and negative. This makes everyone feel insecure about the future. But people with a disability are now in the open like never before, and they are better supported than ever before. It is a federal scheme, so the funding is mainstreamed. And although it is a big social change, the outcome will be positive.

In addition to NDIS, there are also sporting groups that can help with people who have a disability (for example, Gymnastics Australia has a fantastic, inclusive program,[21] as does Triathlon Australia[22]). Many local swimming pools now have programs for kids with disabilities. There is a long history of support programs for athletics (for example, in preparation for the Paralympics).

Now we can see people with a disability more engaged with our community. They are less likely to be sitting at home with little care or few supports.

Physical activity clubs and social groups are engaging with people with a disability to support them. It is becoming more likely that work environments will include an increasing number of the disabled population. The outcome for Australian society will be a positive one.

---

21   gymnastics.org.au/GA/Gymsports/Gymnastics_for_All/Gymability/ Shared_Content/Gymsports/GfA/Gymability.aspx

22   triathlon.org.au/Para_Tri/People_with_Disabilities

Chapter Nine

The Importance of Preventative Care and Community Support

Australia is a proud nation. Its people tend to be direct and laid back, culturally speaking. However, many Australians do not view asking for help as a good thing. It goes against our nature to have to place ourselves at the mercy of someone else.

As a nation, we pride ourselves on being inventive and able to manage several different tasks independently. We are very individualistic and stoic, and these are considered positive traits in our behaviour. Most of the time, this is a good thing.

But it provides a challenge when it comes to healthcare. Preventative care is cheaper and improves our quality of life. However, we think it is a strength to try to manage our own needs without speaking to others, even when we are not sure about something. (I realise this makes us sound quite similar across the nation, but we are not—there are some communities that understand that humbling yourself and asking for help is in fact a strength.)

When we consider our health, Australians need to learn the art of asking for help earlier. If your body is telling you something is wrong, go see a GP.

Trusting your GP is important. They are knowledgeable about health and can often identify a problem early, before you end up in hospital.

If your car was making a funny noise, you would take it to a mechanic to fix—especially if it was something you could not easily figure out. The same goes for caring for your body.

We are a sporting nation and running our bodies hard is common. Occasionally, we need to have a check-up. Getting in early reduces the risk of something more serious developing that will require more invasive care and support later on.

Therefore, primary healthcare needs to be more available and held in higher esteem. It is hard to sell to the community, though.

The importance of community support.

Preventative care means that nothing is actually wrong or that chronic disease is well-managed. The concept of preventing a health issue is confusing to many. We are getting better at it, but it continues to be a challenge for people to understand.

Why should we pay for something we do not need?

Community services have developed piecemeal—that is, only as things are thought to be needed. As discussed earlier, there was not much help in the community prior to the 1970s for people to manage their health. GPs and nurses (through RDNS) were expected to provide home care and manage chronic conditions. They were quite capable of performing these tasks, but it was an expensive and unregulated practice. Many families looked after their sick family member at home. So, in the 1970s, community health services were set up to provide supportive care to people nearer their homes.

Different programs were designed in response to the needs of the local community. As a result, health services in different communities provided different programs. Over time, community health services merged and other organisations started to compete for their funds. In addition, advocacy groups and philanthropic organisations began offering new programs.

Therefore, the complexity of community health services increased and referring people to their programs has become challenging for even the most experienced healthcare professionals.

Taking the time to get to know your GP allows them to assess when further interactions with community health services are required. A GP will usually have an understanding of who they can confidently direct their patients to.

**Gary's medication misunderstanding
led him to be hospitalised several times.**

His GP referred him to RDNS and they were able
to help Gary understand his medication regimen
and improve his lifestyle.

A GP was having a hard time with Gary, one of his patients. Gary had been diagnosed with Chronic Obstructive Pulmonary Disease (COPD) and he required daily medications to manage the condition. But every couple of months, Gary ended up in hospital with pneumonia.

The GP did not know why this was happening but wanted Gary to have a better quality of life. Gary's pulmonary condition was so bad that he was already living in a wheelchair.

In frustration, the GP called Helen, a nurse working with RDNS, and asked her to visit Gary at home and find out what was happening.

After a few visits, Helen established that Gary stopped his preventative medications whenever he felt well. He could not see the point of taking medication while he was well. Unfortunately, each time this happened he would end up in hospital.

Helen attempted to explain the medications to Gary and why he needed to keep taking them. Gary, however, remained unconvinced. He kept stopping his medications and ending up back in hospital. His health deteriorated to the extent that he was no longer able to walk his dog—they used to go out to the local park each day, with Gary in his wheelchair and the dog walking beside him.

Over time, though, Helen found out Gary liked to gamble. He loved horse racing and trying his luck on Tattersalls. One day, Helen said to Gary, 'Prove me wrong'. He had stopped his medications again, and she was sure this meant he would end up in hospital once more.

Helen said, 'Take your medications as the doctor prescribed, and if you end up in hospital again, then you can tell me, "I told you so"'.

He did not go to hospital after that for a few years. In fact, he started to walk his dog again, which was what he loved to do.

Helen also connected Gary to the local community health service and organised regular cleanings and Meals on Wheels for him.

His quality of life improved dramatically as a result.

Community health services are a major provider of allied health services, such as physiotherapy, occupational therapy, speech therapy, counselling, mental health, and drug and alcohol treatment services. The funding of these services was inconsistent and led many programs to be developed and then closed or changed. This, in turn, led to many community health services finding it difficult to provide a holistic program for their patients.

The smaller community health groups have struggled to stay afloat and have been absorbed by the larger services. Mental health programs are the most difficult to fund but are increasingly required.

Tracey's mental health problems led to family breakdown and ongoing lifestyle problems for her.

Eventually, getting the right help improved her circumstances.

Tracey married early and had three children. She did not finish high school, but her husband Steve was a good provider.

After her third child, Tracey struggled to manage the household chores and stick within the household budget. She found it hard to concentrate and things were getting her down. She then stopped seeing her high school friends.

Her husband was working long hours and would often come home after she had gone to bed. Tracey became lonely. She just could not deal with her children's constant neediness.

She went to her local GP to see if he could give her something to help her concentrate. He could not find anything wrong, but she did seem down. He referred her to the local maternal and child health nurse for support.

Eventually, Tracey started having a couple of glasses of wine each night to help her sleep. She never saw the maternal and child health nurse because the last time she had gone to the nurse's clinic, the long wait had made her children bored and unmanageable.

Tracey and Steve began arguing because of his absence. This cycle became insidious, and Tracey's drinking increased.

One day, a neighbour found the children playing on the road and could not find Tracey anywhere. When Steve came home from work, he found Tracey asleep in one of the children's beds. Child Protection Services were called and Tracey was sent to a drug and alcohol clinic.

Steve had had enough and separated from Tracey. With his new girlfriend, he took custody of the children.

Tracey was eventually discharged from the drug and alcohol clinic and returned home. She was monitored periodically, but was also expected to make the effort to go to her regular appointments with a drug and alcohol counsellor.

The counsellor tried to get her to attend some programs that the community health service provided, but Tracey felt uncomfortable in a group setting.

She became increasingly isolated. She saw her children rarely, as Steve kept taking them away on holidays.

Tracey continued to struggle to concentrate, so getting a job was difficult, and she eventually went back to her GP. They talked for a long time and the GP wondered if Tracey had postnatal depression. He sent her to see a psychiatrist for diagnosis. The GP organised the appointment and rang Tracey to make sure she went.

The psychiatrist confirmed the diagnosis and changed Tracey's medications. With further counselling through the community health service, as well as time, Tracey started feeling like her old self. She joined a gym and became a personal trainer. She now sees her children more regularly and is working again.

Tracey was lucky she kept seeing her regular GP. He was able to help her to get better. But the path to getting better was not straightforward, and her family broke up because of it.

She was also lucky to live in the city, as these services are much harder to access in the country.

Healthcare policy now recognises that community health services should be at the forefront of primary and preventative care initiatives. Ideally, we need to fund community health services properly so they can deliver quality primary care at the local level. This will support people close to where they live.

Community health services serve a fundamental role in innovative and integrated responses to primary care, comprehensive preventative health programs, and health promotion activities. Understanding the nature of the community the services are being offered in is central to good outcomes.

We also need collaborative partnerships within the local community to provide unique responses to both healthcare and health promotion. A supportive community health service, which is engaged and has strong ties locally, ensures that healthcare is aligned with the needs of the area.

Providing the community with a single point of contact is an essential element of supporting individualised healthcare. As we have seen, this is not currently how it is done. Patients need to search for the right community health service for their primary healthcare, which makes the task frustrating and limiting.

Community health services have core components of health service provision, and also the ability to adapt and respond to locally identified health gaps and funding opportunities. Partnership and local responsiveness is a feature of community health, which is the natural home of quality primary healthcare and service delivery.

Community health services also need to work in a capacity that ensures transparency and accountability to the local community. This occurs when services are locally situated and engage in purposeful relationships with other organisations in the area.

Community development principles are universally based on social justice, fairness, empowerment, partnership, community involvement and participation. The lower the person's health status, the less likely they are to fully participate in society.

Overcoming these barriers is a clear part of the role of community health services.

Funding for community health and holistic approaches to health and wellbeing need to be considered more fully by our policy makers. This will ensure an increased focus on prevention, community, care in the home and, perhaps most importantly, access to services close to home.

The role of community health services is to deliver more comprehensive, preventative health programs. This points to a shared vision between the state and territory governments and local community health, and a reinforcement of the principles of community healthcare.

In this environment and with this shared vision, community health and the acute sector need to form a true partnership, founded on mutual respect.

We need to develop programs and initiatives that reduce the pressure on hospital services. We should consider whether some acute programs might be better managed in the community setting as opposed to free resources in the hospital environment. Healthcare coaching will also support this premise and ensure people are cared for more effectively within their own home.

Between community health provision and the acute sector, we need to look critically at chronic disease to identify and develop community-based responses that will reduce presentation admissions and readmissions to hospital. This essentially involves finding ways to connect the management of an individual's complex health needs across a continuum of services in hospital, rehabilitation, residential and community settings.

Every healthcare provider needs to encourage and support incorporating early intervention and prevention into all aspects of healthcare and daily life. Nowhere is this more urgent than with people suffering from a mental illness. About 70% of adult mental health problems emerge before the age of 25. An estimated 45% of Australians aged 16–85 will experience a mental health disorder during their lifetime.

Early intervention is the key. Finding ways to reduce risk and prevent the development of chronic mental illness is critical.

The combination of mental health problems and alcohol and drug abuse is common. People with mental health disorders also have a much higher rate of severe disability and a lower life expectancy than those without them.

Engagement with the community is important to encourage individual health and wellbeing. To successfully build on the current systems, we also need to embrace diversity, respect specific expertise, recognise areas of specialty, and accept limitations within the medical system.

The establishment of a healthcare coaching role that utilises experienced community health professionals within GP's practices and in hospital wards would be invaluable. Healthcare coaches can provide experienced health and wellbeing assessments, and provide active assistance in referring patients appropriately into the community. They would also be adept at explaining medical diagnoses and supporting people through the transitions from and to health.

Ultimately, having experienced healthcare coaches to assist patients will reduce readmissions into the acute sector. That means, we reduce the waste of taxpayers' money. When patients are readmitted to the hospital, the impact on them is often dramatic and these negative effects generally flow on to their loved ones.

Gaining a greater awareness of the community environment leads to a greater understanding of the community and the management of an individual's health and wellbeing. By developing relationships and aligning the health system closer to the community, we can support proactive community development. Understanding the population and its health needs means we can respond in the way that the community wants.

We need to consider the challenges people face in primary healthcare. We need to engage individuals and their families at the points where they are at their most vulnerable. We need to support them through the complexity of the Australian healthcare system.

This is where the transitions between acute and primary care in the community must be supported.

Chapter Ten

The Problems of Mental Health Policy

When the British first colonised Australia in 1788, they jailed the mentally ill with criminals. Twenty years later, they established asylums for the mentally ill. This system persisted until the late 1980s, when the governments of the day, in their wisdom, closed these asylums so the mentally ill could be managed in the community. However, they barely considered how this care would be delivered to the newly released patients. The consequences for many of these people have been disastrous. Numerous have ended up homeless, while others have been imprisoned.

Australia now has two separate medical systems. The first is for those who are physically ill, while the second is for the mentally ill. Coordination between these systems is minimal, particularly in acute settings such as hospitals. If a person is having an acute crisis that combines mental and physical conditions, there are no facilities that can treat both conditions properly.

Someone with a known mental health condition who is suffering a psychotic episode often cannot connect with their doctors until they have been admitted to a secure mental health ward. These mental health wards cannot deal with physical illness. If the patient subsequently develops a medical condition, such as pneumonia, they are typically transferred to a general ward in a medical hospital until the physical condition is resolved.

Therefore, the mentally ill patient finds themselves in a general ward, which cannot manage their mental health. If their physical health improves, they are often discharged like a normal patient instead of being returned to the secure ward to resolve their mental health condition. Once in a nonsecure ward, they can discharge themselves to the community. Patients may do this if they have previously had a negative experience in a secure ward, which has left them understandably afraid to return. Self-discharge by the patient forces their family to deal with a psychotic person without community support.

In general, families struggle to deal with such crises. They often flounder while trying to find help. Community services that might assist them are already stretched to their maximum. Even when these services can help, it could be days or even weeks before they are able to do so—long enough for something terrible to happen. At this point, the mentally ill often become homeless or fall into the grip of the criminal justice system.

Mark's deteriorating mental health combined with a physical ailment led to inadequate care

Getting police involved
was the best thing that happened
(a statement you would not normally hear).

Mark was a middle-aged family man who was diagnosed with schizophrenia in his early twenties. In recent times, he had lost his job as a labourer. Being the main breadwinner for his wife and children and taking pride in that role of provider, the loss of self-worth exacerbated his schizophrenia.

As his condition worsened, Mark was admitted to a secure ward in a Melbourne public hospital. These wards are often considered unpleasant places, and he would have done anything to get out of it. While there, Mark was getting his normal psychiatric treatment to stabilise his psychosis. He was also being seen by a GP on the ward when possible, and this GP diagnosed him with severe pneumonia. Mark was immediately transferred to the hospital's emergency department for treatment.

The severity of his pneumonia meant that Mark spent several days in the hospital's intensive care unit. Once recovered, he was transferred to a general ward in the hospital for a couple of days. At this point, his wife advocated on the family's behalf that he should be returned to the secure ward to finish his psychiatric treatment.

Instead, Mark was discharged to a rehabilitation center. Because it was not a secure ward, he was able to discharge himself, which is exactly what he did.

Once home, Mark initially refused to see his GP. His family was able to change his mind, however. Mark was still going through his psychotic episode when he saw his GP, but the GP nonetheless thought Mark would be safe in his family's care.

The family tried their best to care for Mark at home while waiting for support from community services.

At this stage, he had become severely paranoid. He thought people were chasing him. He was not sleeping and would run around the streets at night and get lost.

His family was very distraught.

Mark even tried to burn his house down, as he believed someone was going through his private information. His paranoia made him aggressive, and he struck his wife, even though he was normally a very passive and kind man who would only rarely raise his voice, let alone become physically aggressive.

His family had to try to provide 24-hour care for Mark until somebody came to help. In the end, it was the police who were able to do this.

He actually asked the police to take him to a safe place, so they returned him to the secure ward. Mark's paranoia probably saved his life.

The family had become terrified that he would hurt himself. Mark was still recovering from the pneumonia, but he needed to be in a secure ward to get the person-centred care he needed.

Unfortunately, because of how the system currently works, the treatments you would normally provide to someone with pneumonia, such as physiotherapy, speech therapy or treatment by a specialist respiratory nurse—all of which would have happened in a general rehabilitation ward—could not be offered to Mark in the secure ward. He was treated for two different conditions in two different situations. As a result, both conditions received inadequate treatment, which caused unnecessary suffering for both Mark and his family.

No matter what his wife advocated for to support the family, the health system structure does not enable any integration between the mental and the medical. No crossover was allowed. Conditions that should have been treated simultaneously—after all, it is about the whole body!—were unnecessarily separated. There was no process within the system to allow for parallel treatments. It was left to the family to coordinate Mark's medical care.

This separation of care put a lot of pressure on Mark's family to manage, especially when he had two serious conditions that could have killed him. The family's fears were real and justified. They had been left to manage Mark's condition without support.

In the end, Mark stabilised, went home, and was okay. The community nurse saw him for a time. Things settled down. The outcome was positive, but not without a lot of unwanted work and stress on the family that should not have happened.

Australia needs to trial a program that situates high-dependency beds within a small number of mental health wards, with medical staff and allied health workers who can treat patients' medical conditions alongside the usual psychiatric staff to provide the treatment needed to manage someone suffering a psychotic episode.

What should we do next? What should we do to move forward with this?

We advance by providing high-dependency care units within the system, whether in medical hospitals or in the mental health area, that gives us the ability to ensure that patients' mental and medical needs are both being looked after. Staff can be trained to work in those areas, to understand the difficulties they might come across.

There needs to be more understanding about how a mental health crisis, such as the one in the case study, affects the family as well as the patient. The patient has complex needs, and the patient's family are talking to a person—the patient—whom they do not recognise, and who is also unwell.

Treating professionals cannot reason with mentally ill patients like they would any other person. They have to be able to adapt to the patient's needs and understand their journey. That should not be the place of the family. It should be the place of trained staff who support the family through such a time.

We have some very well-trained medical and allied health staff. In city hospitals at least, we have the physical space to set up high-dependency care beds distinct from intensive care beds.

Psychotic behaviour is unlikely to occur in intensive care wards, as the patient is too sick. In a high-dependency unit, however, the person would be well enough to assess their mental as well as physical health accurately. Victoria has already had some discussion about this sort of work. We need to press ahead with it. The distress we see in the community is already too high.

It is difficult for somebody with a mental health condition to function safely in the community. Many people use drugs or steal things because they cannot afford basic necessities and may struggle to manage their own finances or home due to their mental state.

We do not prioritise mental health enough. Too many people are dying by suicide, and there are disproportionate numbers of people with mental health needs in our jails.

The right level of community support and the ability for families to advocate for their loved ones without being dismissed is fundamental to providing better care for the mentally ill in Australia. This is not easy. It will be difficult and expensive to initiate, but when the long-term benefits of prevention are considered, it becomes an imperative.

Australia has a fantastic public healthcare system. There are, however, gaps in the system that require addressing. I believe a lot of people would like to see that happen. We need to give mental health services the funding it deserves, send petitions to all levels of government advocating for change, and hound our leaders to improve support for this community.

Chapter Eleven

The Hurdle is Asking for Help

Current gaps in our healthcare system increasingly leave people in social isolation, unable to manage their home and relationships. These people are struggling to manage their health needs, which means they repeatedly end up in hospital and become increasingly disabled.

The confusing nature of different healthcare services means that individuals who need help may not be referred to the right service.

Why is there such confusion across the healthcare system? We discussed earlier the varied nature of funding across the community healthcare services. This has meant that services have developed differently and referral pathways have become confusing. When you are in hospital, they often treat you for the issue you came in for without much consideration for the other conditions you may have, the impact of the new condition on your life, and what happens when you go home.

Many people find a new diagnosis frightening and do not fully understand the complexities of treatments or ongoing care requirements. There are also people who never manage to find funds or services since they do not fit into the strict acceptance criteria for assistance programs, or who become disillusioned and feel like they do not deserve to be supported.

Oftentimes, when people are not managing their healthcare, it's due to the complexities within our system, particularly where there is a transition from hospital to home. These individuals have 'fallen through the cracks'. It doesn't help that people find it hard to keep asking for help. (It is not the Australian way.) But not asking for help can be a barrier to getting the right support.

Rachel's need for support in the home is only identified by a friend.

Rachel has a chronic condition called 'juvenile diabetes' (now known as 'Type 1 diabetes'). Her diabetes is not well-controlled, despite many trips to the hospital. She commonly has very low blood sugar, which causes her to have seizures.

Her husband has severe depression and has trouble even getting out of bed. He is quite unwell.

They also have two young children. Rachel struggles to manage work and the house. But she is young and appears quite capable, so when she is discharged from hospital, no one thinks to offer her support at home.

More recently, Rachel has started to have trouble with severe asthma, so her trips to hospital have become more regular. She was really struggling and becoming increasingly socially isolated.

An old friend, David, rang her to see how she was going. She opened up to him and said that she was floundering. She was struggling to maintain employment and manage the household. David worked in local government in the town planning department. He knew that his local council had services that could help his friend.

He rang them for her and was reassured that they could help. He rang Rachel back and gave her the number to call. She was able to get help with home cleaning and Meals on Wheels.

Rachel could not believe the difference this made for her family. Her medical needs were still concerning, but at least her family life was more stable. She was lucky to have a friend like David; otherwise, she would have continued to struggle.

She did not know that she could ask for help from the local council, nor did she think she could even if it was an option. But in talking with David, he gave her the permission she needed to seek help. Despite her constant contact with hospital and medical services, no one had realised that she was struggling and needed this assistance.

Early in my career as a young nurse, I worked in the orthopaedic ward of a large city hospital. As a new graduate, I had little knowledge of what was available in the community. I also had little understanding of what was needed for people when they were discharged.

My job was to manage the patient's healthcare until discharge and then I thought they would go to their GP for community support. The hospital had a social work department for patients with complex needs at home, but there were only two social workers for the whole hospital, so referral to them was restricted. It often delayed a hospital discharge as well, so it was typically discouraged. This was what I experienced and is commonly the perspective of nurses in the hospital.

As I soon found out, people were not getting the support they needed on discharge. Their GP was often not in a position to refer them to community services because they did not know what was available. To make matters worse, GPs do not always know when their patient has been discharged from hospital. Unfortunately, communication between the GP and the hospital continues to need work.

A GP will often refer patients to RDNS if there are concerns about medications or wounds that need regular dressing. This would then lead to further referrals to community services. Most nurses working in RDNS are fully aware of what services are available for people, and they visit individuals in their homes so they can see what support is needed.

But many people who are discharged from hospital do not go to their GP routinely and never get referred on to services in the community. How would they know on their own what services are available for them, and who is responsible for telling them? What can we do to improve things now without it costing a huge amount?

Health literacy is a problem for many patients with a new medical diagnosis. This can only be resolved by effective communication with a healthcare professional.

Because of the current restrictive funding options and time constraints, patients are given little time with their GP in which to understand their diagnosis. Often, but not always, the GP will provide their patient with some written information about their new diagnosis and treatment regimen. Then the patients go home and find they have forgotten half of what the GP told them, as well as significant parts of the treatment regimen. This is very common, as patients are rarely health literate and are usually distressed and in pain.

This then becomes a real issue. If patients do not follow the directions the GP has given them, they may end up in hospital.

Due to the medical illness they see their GP about, they may be referred to a specialist. The waiting times and the cost of seeing a specialist can be daunting. If the referral goes into the public system, it can take several months to a year to wait for an outpatient appointment. Sometimes, the referral letter gets lost, so no appointment is ever made. People become disillusioned and feel that they are being left stranded. They try to keep managing with their condition, but without the treatment they need to overcome it.

Having a supportive community health nurse or other healthcare contact (like a coach) will mean that the average person can get the follow-up care they need. A supportive coach can help guide the person through the healthcare system. They can provide detailed explanations and supportive community or welfare information if a patient thinks of a question after seeing their GP. The coach can follow up on referrals and ensure that the recommendations of the GP are followed.

This would provide the patient with better service and aid GPs in their practice. The role of a coach would be quite separate from that of a practice nurse, as the coach would have no clinical responsibility. They would be there to provide support and guidance.

Ideally, a coach would see the patient in the GP's offices before they go in to see the GP. The coach can ask questions and have the patient's home needs assessed. This enables the GP to have as much information as possible. Then, after the GP has met with the patient, the coach can answer questions about services and make referrals, which provides time for the patient to ask questions and get the additional support they need.

Many people search the internet for more information about their diagnosis. If they don't know where to look or don't understand the information the search has provided, they may get confused or even more worried.

There are some great websites available in Australia with information about common medical conditions.

For example, the Australian National Health and Medical Research Council (NHMRC) has set up the Better Health Channel.[23] The NHMRC provides well-researched and easily understood health information that is also translated into several commonly used languages.

There are also some excellent advisory services that can provide support for people with a chronic medical condition or disability.

Beyondblue[24] is an organisation that provides information and support to people with mental health issues. People with severe depression often end up isolated and unsupported because their loved ones don't know how to help them or how to deal with the constant negativity. Beyondblue can provide support on the phone or recommend a group or service that can help the person manage their depression. They have had a lot of success in helping people with mental health issues.

Philanthropic organisations, such as the Rotary or Lions clubs, also provide a wide range of services and equipment that would otherwise not be available to people.

Families often pay for services and equipment to support a family member who is unwell, such as setting up medical devices at home so their loved one can remain there. A wife who develops multiple sclerosis (MS) is a possible example. Her MS may worsen to the point that she is increasingly unable to

---

23   betterhealth.vic.gov.au

24   beyondblue.org.au

move and requires special equipment to manage at home. The government may subsidise some equipment, but it will not necessarily subsidise all the equipment that her husband believes he needs to help her stay at home. He wants her to be with him and refuses to let her go into care. He is also getting older and requires extensive support to manage her and keep her in the family home.

Some philanthropic organisations will help if you need a wheelchair or need to install a motorised stairwell chair. Other philanthropic organisations have a preferred condition or medical service they provide funding for.

Federal and state governments will cover many items, but not everything. If a person requires a certain level of care or needs a treatment that has not been approved, the government will not provide monetary support.

A further issue is how long it takes to get the help you need. This is the hole that philanthropic organisations can fill, if only people knew who to ask for the help they need.

Chapter Twelve

The Relevance of Healthcare Assessments

Healthcare professionals need to be more account- able for their evaluations. A holistic approach to health examinations is essential for making an appropriate diagnosis and treatment plan.

Active listening takes place when you, as the audi- ence, are paying full attention to the speaker, not only with your ears but also with your eyes and your mind. This becomes hard when you are hearing similar stories repeatedly, where the only difference is the person who has walked through the door.

As part of the assessment, the healthcare provider or doctor will also need to engage with the new patient and interpret their body language. The healthcare professional needs to verify what they have heard by asking questions to reduce the possibility of making assumptions. Again, making assumptions is easy to do when you have heard similar stories before.

There are many people in the healthcare profession who do this well. However, it is often hard to get in for an appointment with them.

Providing a holistic assessment requires that the health professional is paying attention to what may be different this time.

Like anyone else, GPs and specialists can become complacent. They see many people with similar conditions, so they can start to assume they know what needs to be done. There is a sense that most people are much the same.

Research and years of study also provide them with an educational standard on which to base their knowledge. But making a good assessment requires that they consider the person in front of them and understand their patient's individual circumstances. Most issues occur when communication is not clear. Asking the right questions and actively listening to the answers is a simple risk management tool for any healthcare provider.

The person meeting with the medical professional may be the exception to the rule, not a textbook case. Healthcare providers can miss this, especially if their knowledge is highly specialised. The last two hundred people they saw were standard textbook cases, so they can easily miss the one who doesn't fit the rule. They might not ask the right questions or make a full physical assessment because they feel, often unconsciously, that they have seen this before.

This is how major medical errors occur—and media attention often follows. Reputations are affected and healthcare services lose funding. Healthcare professionals can lose their registration to practice and possibly go to jail or be fined.

Unfortunately, the people affected the most are usually the people who received inadequate medical treatment. They can suffer lifelong disabilities or, worse, die as a result. The subsequent effect on the family is also significant.

The serious effect of a health professional's inadequate assessment.

A new mother, Sally, pregnant with her first child, was told to have an elective caesarean by her obstetrician because she had previously had surgery on her uterus that put her at risk of bleeding during childbirth. On the day of the surgery, the anaesthetist saw the mother for the first time. Earlier appointments had been cancelled because the anaesthetist was too busy.

The anaesthetist asked Sally if she would like spinal or general anaesthetic. Since Sally had back problems, she was worried that the spinal anaesthetic would not work, so asked for the general.

Her back problems had caused her to stop work and made the pregnancy difficult. Her husband Bill had to take time off work during the final months of the pregnancy because she could not manage without help.

Sally was coerced by the anaesthetist into having the spinal anaesthesia, as this would help with breastfeeding. It would also mean that her husband could watch the surgery.

Without further discussion about her back problems and because she wanted to do the right thing, Sally agreed to the spinal. Five minutes into the surgery, the anaesthetic stopped working.

It took five hours for the pain to be controlled enough for Sally to finally see her child. Because she required significant pain relief, she could not breastfeed for twenty-four hours.

So, the shortened assessment by the anaesthetist significantly impaired Sally's ability to breastfeed and Sally was so distraught by the experience she and her husband both thought she would die.

After three weeks of trying to breastfeed and the development of recurrent infections in her breasts, Sally decided to bottle-feed.

Several months later, Sally was diagnosed with post-traumatic stress disorder (PTSD). It took another several months of regular psychology appointments and treatment for Sally to feel safe again.

Bill had taken time off to care for Sally and their little girl. This had an impact on his work. He also took a long time to recover from the ordeal.

Another health practitioner who knew Sally told her, in a social setting, that because she had a small neural tube defect, a spinal anaesthetic would therefore have simply seeped out of the spine. That is, it would never have lasted. A general anaesthetic would have been more appropriate. The original anaesthetist did not even ask what the new mother's back condition was.

As mentioned earlier, communication is the most important aspect of a good health assessment. Patients are vulnerable and trust that their doctor will ensure that the right treatment is prescribed for them.

The key to a carefully considered treatment plan is a comprehensive and thorough assessment. However, the questions asked may often seem similar to those asked in a previous healthcare professional's assessment and this can be frustrating for patients when they are feeling unwell. Yet this is an essential aspect of providing good care. A good health assessment requires adequate time and should not be rushed unnecessarily. A rushed assessment will, almost certainly, miss crucial information.

In the case study above, Sally told the anaesthetist she had a lot of back problems. This should have alerted the anaesthetist to the possibility that a spinal anaesthetic might not work. With an appropriate amount of time, the anaesthetist might have asked Sally more probing questions about her back problems to decide whether a general anaesthetic should be used in her case.

Taking the time to fully understand a patient's history helps ensure that risks are carefully considered and potentially reduced. Healthcare professionals that provide a holistic and thorough health assessment are not only going to be less likely to make a mistake with the care they provide, they will often be well-regarded by their patient.

However, the healthcare system in Australia is currently understaffed and this makes the potential for mistakes higher. Medical practitioners are rushing and patients often feel isolated and unheard. Streamlining care is not safe or economical. At best, patients lose confidence in the system and look elsewhere for help. At worst, patients die or are permanently disabled. The healthcare system then looks to find new ways to reduce risk, without considering the need for better patient care.

Yet if there were more people trained as healthcare coaches and if sufficient funding existed for them, these coaches would be able to give patients space to express their concerns, allowing them time to consider what they have been told and to ask questions.

Part of their role would be to ensure that the patient's expectations were managed and to facilitate communication between the person receiving care and the healthcare professional responsible for treating them, as well as between healthcare professionals attending to the same individual. These coaches would ensure that patients understand what is being asked of them and support them to access the right treatment and help they need to heal and return to their life safely.

Healthcare coaches would not be doing anyone else's job. They would simply be serving a specialized function, filling a gap that is steadily getting wider due to the evolution of our healthcare system.

Chapter Thirteen

When Medicine Lacks Answers

Specialists have extensive knowledge and experience in a particular area of medicine. They are well-respected and can identify conditions thanks to an intuition developed through their extensive education and experience.

Doctors are highly specialised. Most of the time, a medical specialist is right about the diagnosis and treatment of their patients.

A patient, on the other hand, is vulnerable and worried. They are seeing the specialist because they have a medical condition that is causing illness and pain. They are often stressed, and so is their family.

If the medical specialist cannot find a reason for the symptoms, they can either refer the patient to another specialist or, if they believe the patient is exhibiting signs of psychological distress, refer them for psychiatric assessment and treatment.

The patient is often distressed by their illness and in pain. However, in my experience, patients deal with their distress differently. Some become upset and cry, others get angry, and still others show no emotion at all. I also know of people who put on a brave face, but then become distressed when they reach the safety of their home.

A negative term for a patient who is not considered to be unwell and is exhibiting distress is a 'malingerer'. Historically, there have been several diagnoses for these patients: hysteria, chronic fatigue and, more recently, conversion disorder.

These patients are viewed as either having made up their symptoms or having symptoms that are the result of stress. Sometimes, this is true. Munchausen's Syndrome is a classic psychiatric diagnosis of a patient who is trying to gain sympathy from others by either making up symptoms of a medical condition or hurting themselves to mimic a medical syndrome.

However, this is rare. Sometimes, medical understanding hasn't developed enough to effectively diagnose a condition. Medical technology has not caught up.

Chronic fatigue syndrome is a classic example of how the knowledge to accurately diagnose a medical condition was lacking. In the 1990s, chronic fatigue syndrome was often the diagnosis given to patients when another cause could not be established. Patients were presenting with extreme fatigue and often had intermittent fevers and sinus congestion.

As research into chronic fatigue continued, however, it established better testing techniques. Now, people are often diagnosed with post-viral syndrome, which happens after a serious viral condition such as glandular fever. There is also now a blood test that determines if someone has diagnosable chronic fatigue syndrome.

Currently, when a medical specialist cannot diagnose a condition, patients are given the psychiatric diagnosis of 'conversion disorder'. This is a medical condition that was described by psychiatrists treating patients who had stopped being able to walk or move their limbs after the trauma of war.

Psychiatrists often saw female Vietnamese patients with this syndrome after the Vietnam war. These women were significantly traumatised by seeing people dying, and many had been raped by soldiers. It sounds ludicrous, but patients with medical symptoms, often women in pain or with a movement disorder, are now diagnosed with conversion disorder. However, specialists know that the reason for the medical condition is trauma, and so the patient is referred to a psychiatrist for ongoing treatment.

This occurs instead of the medical specialist just saying they don't know why the patient has this condition. If they humbly admitted they didn't know the cause, and then just treated the symptoms until medical knowledge caught up, I believe many patients would understand.

Patients are being treated for a psychiatric illness unnecessarily. I have heard people comment, 'I am being treated for a trauma in my childhood that I did not know happened.'

Again, most of the people diagnosed with these conditions are women.

**Stacey's diagnosis was missed
because modern technology
wasn't mature enough yet.**

Stacey had left-eye blindness. She was told by the eye specialist that it was not possible for her to be unable to see, and spent most of her life wondering why she couldn't. As it turned out, her optic nerve had not developed properly and the technology of the day simply wasn't able to assess this.

Stacey, a toddler, was falling over a lot, so her mother, Grace, took her to see an eye specialist. Grace was concerned there was something terribly wrong. Stacey's falls were inconsistent with her development, and she was diagnosed with a vision impairment in her left eye.

The ophthalmologist could not see a reason for the vision impairment. However, Stacey had a turned eye, and he thought that might have something to do with it. So, he performed surgery on her left eye to straighten it.

Grace had two other children and a fourth on the way. She was struggling to manage. The most difficult time was when Stacey and her older brother James had the same surgery together. Being pregnant and caring for two young children after these surgeries was hard. Grace also had to manage the rehabilitation of her children after surgery, as there was no one who could help.

Stacey continued having trouble seeing out of her left eye. Her parents were both concerned, so they continued the treatments provided by the specialist. After Stacey's fifth surgery, the specialist was convinced that Grace was not implementing enough of the exercises she had been given that were to help Stacey regain her sight. Grace was heartbroken and left feeling it was her fault.

After several operations and ongoing rehabilitation, Stacey still could not see out of her left eye. The specialist told her mother to continue the rehabilitation treatment. However, Stacey's vision showed no further improvement, which left her family feeling that they had not done enough to help her. The specialist simply did not believe the child could not see.

As she grew up, Stacey still could not see out of her left eye. It had not stopped her doing much, and she was able to do very well in her chosen sport of gymnastics. She also did well at school and went to university.

As an adult, she had further surgery on her eye, which did not improve her vision. The more recent specialist still could not make sense of why Stacey could not see.

Eventually, Stacey started to have problems with her right eye. She went to another specialist. She looked at both eyes. By now, medical technology had improved and the examination was more accurate.

The new specialist could see the nerves behind the eye. They could see that the nerve of Stacey's left eye had not developed fully. Finally, after forty years, medical technology had caught up with what was happening symptomatically with Stacey.

Grace was relieved to know she was not at fault for Stacey's left eye not improving when her daughter was still a child.

It is important to remember that this can still happen today. We have come very far in medical science, but we have not discovered all the answers. There remain diseases and conditions that cannot yet be detected or understood.

Chapter Fourteen

Improving Patient Care and Reducing the Risk of 'Falling through the Gaps'

One of the most common topics of discussion in healthcare is, how do we 'fill the gaps'? How do we improve the transition between hospital and the home?

The Australian state and territory governments have set up numerous projects or programs attempting to improve this transition and reduce readmission to hospital, but these have changed or moved from the community into the hospital.

This alters the ability of patients to access these programs. Referrals continue to rely heavily on nursing staff to know what is available and who can access the programs.

Earlier, I discussed the issue of specialisation and how that has had the subsequent effect of healthcare professionals not knowing where to refer a patient.

A healthcare coach needs to have enough of an understanding about a range of programs to provide appropriate and suitable care for their patients.

First, we need to identify the issue. A holistic assessment should pick up problems that the patient needs help with.

Once the issue is identified, we then need to find the most appropriate referral pathway. This is talked about a lot in healthcare circles (in conferences, research programs and healthcare education). Many projects have been developed to look at referral pathways, but they are often not continued. With so much activity in the area, we have to wonder why the problem continues today.

I have worked in this area, and I believe that we are constantly losing experienced and knowledgeable healthcare staff. They have followed a career path that takes them away from the patient's bedside, as it were, because that is where the career opportunities lie.

Why we need to consider healthcare coaching as a way forward.

Federal, state and territory governments should consider the possibility of a consulting role across the health, aged and disability sectors. Healthcare coaches could come from any medical or allied health field. They would simply need the ability to do effective health assessments and have experience with working in the community.

There is currently a nurse practitioner role, but to attain it requires masters-level study (in other words, research away from direct patient care) and clinical experience is also usually taken into account. This program requires further study and research by a nurse, and that means significant time off work. Also, nurse practitioner positions are difficult to attain so many nurses do not apply.

In my nursing career, I have met many nurses who could provide the high level of care and expertise required. I have also worked with allied health professionals who could easily do this work.

If we had a career path that allowed us to continue to work and use our expertise in a useful and meaningful way, I believe we would all benefit: nurses, allied healthcare professionals, patients and the wider community.

There are many excellent clinicians who are no longer registered because they took time away from the clinical environment due to family responsibilities. Yet many of these clinicians would make excellent healthcare coaches. If such a career path existed for them, we would probably lose fewer good people and our patient care would be greatly improved. This role would need to be seen, not in the context of a clinical position, but as a role that is supportive or advisory to the patient.

Attached to wards, a coach could assess each patient who is ready for discharge to ensure they understand what happened during their hospital stay and what they need to do when they return home. This would include making referrals and appointments, if required. Such support would greatly improve upon the current practice of providing a patient with a one-sentence discharge summary, which is largely unreadable anyway.

In addition, having a coach adjacent to a GP would support people in the community before they get to hospital. We currently rely upon websites and an extraordinary number of pamphlets so that individuals can choose their own healthcare pathway. We expect people to navigate their own way through the healthcare system.

I return to our culturally and linguistically diverse community and to those who cannot read because they are illiterate. In Australia, 1% of adults over fifteen years old are illiterate. This means there are approximately 160,000 adults across Australia who cannot read. The rate is even higher for Aborigines and Torres Strait Islanders. How are they supposed to navigate through the healthcare system?

And then there's the number of people who are computer illiterate. Sometimes, finding the right service provider in the community takes an understanding of what is wrong, knowledge about the possible service providers, and time to phone and find the one that will suit the needs of a patient. Currently, it is mostly left to chance.

We need to consider that every person who enters the healthcare environment usually does so against their will. Who chooses to go to the doctor? This means the patient is naturally going to be distressed. These patients are often vulnerable and require clear and supportive information, preferably provided by someone they are familiar with—not the current, very clinical and foreign experience. We have done such a good job of specialising in medicine that gaps in the system are the natural endpoint.

Australia's healthcare system has its flaws and we can improve. First, we need to challenge some of our assumptions. Then we need to question how our system has become so difficult for many to navigate. Healthcare has become isolating, and I believe we can improve a person's journey through it. Utilising an experienced healthcare coach, one who is skilled in the art of assessment and referral, would improve the flow for the patient through the system.

Australia has become adept at caring for a person's condition, but we are not very good at caring for the *person*. This means people end up isolated and vulnerable. We can do better.

Chapter Fifteen

The Final Decision Maker

We must remember that the patient is the CEO of their healthcare. It is the medical professional's responsibility to ensure that the individual has the necessary healthcare information. But the patient must then balance their understanding of the healthcare advice with the knowledge of what their decision means to them both personally and professionally. They are given advice by trusted advisers (doctors) and make decisions based on the advice, even if that decision is simply to follow what the doctor says. Unless there are exceptional circumstances, the patient is the one who makes the decision about their healthcare and who has to deal with the consequences of that decision.

Leadership has been described as 'the behaviour of an individual when directing the activities of a group towards a shared goal'. A challenge in healthcare is that it is difficult for a vulnerable patient to command the qualities that we typically see in leaders. This explains why we have such a variety of case managers and team leaders in health. However, I would argue that in most healthcare contexts, there is a case for making the *patient* the leader of their healthcare team.

A CEO does not know everything about every aspect of their business. They know what the business is trying to achieve and rely on input from people they trust to give them the information they need to make sound business decisions.

Healthcare providers need to present information to people in a way that the person and their family or caregiver understand. We need to prioritise information exchange as an essential part of healthcare. Practitioners need to establish how best to provide information to help those they are treating make well-informed decisions. We need to understand different levels of knowledge and be culturally sensitive.

We need to ensure that the person is presented with clear, concise and accurate information. This information must allow them to consider and plan for the people and pets in their lives, and also for potential work interruptions. Using active listening techniques and asking the patient questions will enable the healthcare provider to ensure the information given has been understood.

There are, of course, times when a decision must be made by the healthcare provider. In emergency situations, time is limited, and so healthcare providers usually cannot stop to ensure things are explained clearly. But usually, we do have time to stop and think about how to present information and to allow the person to make the decisions about their treatment.

When a person makes a healthcare decision, service providers (medical, nursing or allied healthcare staff) need to respect that decision. The person will be making the decision the same way that a CEO might, with an understanding of the full situation they are faced with: the effect on their family and financial situation, and their own ability to deal with past physical illness or trauma. The person may need to take into consideration their social supports, work-related issues, and the impact the decision might have on themselves and their family.

From a governance perspective, a CEO may make a business decision based on the best advice from people they trust (general managers, finance managers, legal advisers, human resource managers, etc.) and a sound knowledge of the business environment. If anything goes wrong, then the person who is accountable has to deal with whatever follows. If someone has given the CEO bad advice, they will be reprimanded or fired.

Though these situations are very different, the impact of a healthcare professional's bad advice can be catastrophic for the person they are advising. Advice needs to be considered carefully. A doctor has very specialised knowledge and it is important that this is respected. But they cannot know the patient's full story and history. So, in a sense, they need to be sure they are giving that person the advice they need to make an informed decision.

If we look back at Sally's situation in Chapter Nine, we see that she expressed concern about the anaesthetist's decision regarding her care. If the anaesthetist had given Sally adequate time to consider her decision by making sure that the appointment happened prior to the surgery, then the advice given may have been quite different.

The same would have been true if the anaesthetist had considered Sally's concern and asked appropriate questions to ensure that Sally did not have an underlying back condition that made her an inappropriate candidate for a spinal anaesthesia. The damage to Sally's life from the failed anaesthesia would have been avoided. As in all things, *prevention* is far more effective in medicine than *cure*.

Working in healthcare each day means that a healthcare provider risks becoming complacent. We give the same advice over and over again, and the more specialised we are, the more likely it is that the advice is similar. Due to this, we may forget there are cases that are statistical anomalies and that every person we see is an individual, making decisions based on their own understanding of what that decision will mean for their life. Not every decision is life or death; more often, it is about how the decision to do something will be better than doing nothing.

The only person who understands this holistically is the person coming to us for advice. The individual will know how a decision about their health will impact them. They will know who else may be affected by the decision. Healthcare professionals are there to give advice and provide the treatment that is decided on by the individual. They generally do not have to live with the consequences of the decision.

There is an ongoing debate in healthcare about who is the healthcare team leader. Medical staff may argue it is them, since they are the most knowledgeable.

Nursing staff may argue it is them, as they are the ones who spend the most time with—and therefore have specialised health knowledge of—the actual patient.

Allied health professionals, such as physiotherapists, occupational therapists, social workers and so on, will argue that it would depend on the needs of the individual.

In any case, the team leader needs to be the person who can assess the impact to the patient's life the most, not just physically or mentally, but personally and professionally as well.

The healthcare team leader needs to be the patient.

My contention is that it should always be the individual themselves who makes decisions regarding their care. Healthcare providers need to prioritise how they advise the individual so that *the patient can make an informed decision*.

Being skilled at assessment is important because it informs healthcare providers about the diagnosis and treatment. It also informs them what information they should give the patient so that the latter can then make an informed decision. In these discussions, healthcare providers often lose sight of who actually makes the decision about the treatment provided.

Healthcare providers also need to give a patient adequate time to consider what they have been told. Often, providers are rushing from one patient to the next—they have other people to see and reports to write. But the patient is typically unwell and distressed, and they may be in pain as well. It is easier to rush a decision about treatment because once a decision is made, the healthcare professional can move on to the treatment. But if we consider the decision-making context, it is clear that a patient may need time.

Healthcare providers need to recognise this and reconsider how we make appointments. It is common for a patient to forget some or even all the information we have given them, or to misinterpret the information. They may need to ask questions more than once before making a decision. If they are allowed to do this, the decision they make will be a more considered one.

As stated earlier, a different situation would arise in an emergency. There is a clear differentiation of responsibility in this context. The smartest person in the room, typically a medical specialist or doctor, will need to be decisive. The decisions will be based on what is considered the most urgent need of the patient—to keep them alive in the best health possible until they can choose a course of treatment themselves. If there is a reason the patient cannot make a decision, then the person doing so for them would be the next of kin—that is, the person with the closest relationship to the patient who has the capability to decide. This comes into the legalities of responsibility, and could be a husband or wife, parent or legal guardian.

Conclusion

Healthcare professionals need to become more comfortable with admitting when they don't know something. Making a referral, or simply saying 'I do not know', is likely to improve your relationship with the patient. People respect those who are able to acknowledge the limits of their knowledge.

The medical profession does not hold the answer to everything that ails us. We have a lot to learn about how the body works. A lot of what we do know is based on a best guess. For example, 'this medicine works for this condition—we do not actually know why, but it works—so we continue to provide the medication and maybe one day we will know how it works.' There are many examples of this, as there is still a lot to learn, and we are learning all the time.

The story of Stacey in Chapter Ten, with her bad eyesight, shows us that we need to consider this in the context of care. Eye specialists thought they knew everything they needed to know about the eye. They were certain that Stacey's problem was due to a turned eye. It took medicine forty years to realise that she actually could not use her left eye because the nerve had not formed properly.

It requires humility to acknowledge that we do not understand everything about the body. Medicine is continuously learning and technology is improving. The more we learn, the more we realise we do not know. We will become proficient in our understanding of human bodies as our techniques for studying them become more refined.

If we have ruled out a possible emotional context to a patient's symptoms, we need to consider asking a different specialist or simply saying we 'do not know' to the patient. If we leave them thinking 'it's in their head' (in other words, it's psychological because we cannot find a reason), this can have a significant damaging impact on them. It can affect their relationships and their work. If a health professional says they do not know, but then treats the patient's symptoms, even pain symptoms, then our patients might trust us more.

The assessment of a patient is the most important risk management process that medicine can carry out. Doctors will meet the patient in different environments, whether in medical rooms, in emergency, on a ward or in the patient's home. The patient may be able to move about freely or they may be in bed. It does not matter where the doctor performs the initial examination; he or she needs to be present and to use active listening techniques to ensure they are getting the answers that will help them make a diagnosis.

Sitting at a desk and looking at a computer means that the doctor will lose a large amount of non-verbal communication. If they are not assessing body language, they are missing a lot.

In addition, just because a patient is in bed when the doctor meets them does not mean they are not able to make informed decisions, or that the medical doctor should not perform a physical examination because it is inconvenient.

Too often, we look at the patients' notes to see what assessments have been performed and diagnoses made, even before we see a patient. It makes the assessment much faster, but if someone has not done an adequate assessment or has made a wrong diagnosis, it means we carry the wrong diagnosis into our evaluation.

Health assessments need to be done as though the patient is quite able to make decisions, even though they may be in a vulnerable state. This will reduce mistakes, and it will also mean the patient will feel they are being listened to. It is when health professionals make assumptions that problems arise.

As an individual, a person needs to be ready for a health crisis. Ideally, we should have a local GP who provides us with guidance regarding health promotion. This means we see the GP if we are changing our health habits, for a check-up, and for feedback on our diet and exercise. We might also see the GP if we require vaccinations for travel or as our family grows. Another possible reason is to check for sunspots. Australians love sun and sport. This is a good thing, but it puts us at risk for skin cancer. A regular check-up with your GP might pick up a problem early and reduce this risk.

Any of us may experience a medical crisis at some stage. Having a relationship with your local GP means there is someone with both detailed medical knowledge and an understanding of your family history. Your local GP will support you through a medical crisis.

Finally, society needs to consider the prospect of using healthcare coaches in understanding and supporting patients through the complexities of the healthcare system. Aligning the coaches with local GPs or in hospitals aligned with wards will mean they are available at the point of a patient's interaction with the healthcare system.

Every patient has a different story. There needs to be a professional who has a distinct understanding of healthcare and welfare systems, and also has experience working in the community. This would provide a more streamlined approach to patients moving through the healthcare system.

Coaches would need to be highly proficient in assessment and knowledgeable in the full healthcare system. This includes the acute, secondary (rehabilitation and long-term care) and community care settings, as well as supportive services, such as Centrelink and philanthropic services.

There are many of these experts in Australia now, but they end up in management, policy or research settings and do not connect with patients. If we are able to entice them to remain in patient settings, we can better support our community.

It would be a more economical option than fixing problems after they occur. This is a social reform that is urgent.

In conclusion, here are the key points to consider:

1. Australia needs to spend more on caring for our community at home rather than in hospital.

2. Health professionals need to become better at assessment and communication.

3. Health professionals need to admit when they do not know what conditions are afflicting a patient and be less ready to ascribe psychological issues to a patient when they are unable to find a reason for their symptoms, especially when it comes to pain management.

4. People need to develop a relationship with their local GP so the GP is better able to tell when they are unwell.

5. Finally, people need to learn to ask for help when they need it. There are many service supports in Australia, but no one can help if people do not ask.

I have had a varied and interesting healthcare career and it is heartbreaking when I come across people who are in need of help, but aren't getting it.

The healthcare system is complex—even those working within it find it challenging to know what is available for people outside their scope of knowledge.

I hope my case studies show you just how complicated it is and help you on your journey.

Thank you for reading *Surviving Healthcare in Australia*. If you've enjoyed reading this book, please leave a review on your favourite review site. It helps me reach more readers who may benefit from the information provided herein.

A Short History of the
Australian Healthcare System

To understand how we got to where we are today, we need to look at the history of Australia's healthcare system. It's only with that understanding that we can find solutions to make it better in the future.

When the system was first implemented, it made sense. But it has become outdated and doesn't reflect modern healthcare needs. There is a gap that's growing and it's forcing medical professionals to raise their rates to the point that many patients can't afford it, even though they've been paying for comprehensive health insurance all along.[25] But to understand how we got here, we need to look at where we've been.

The Australian healthcare system began with medical services provided only to people who could afford to pay or who were covered by charity. As a result, many Australians ended up bankrupt and destitute due to illness. Families gave up everything in order to pay for the care of a loved one. If that person also

---

25   The government has no control over the pricing the medical professionals charge. They do set the subsidies for Medicare, but doctors can charge what they want. Since the government isn't increasing the subsidies, doctors' only option for a pay raise is to increase their rates.

happened to be the main breadwinner, it was even harder for the family to manage financially.

Prior to the introduction of universal healthcare, families had to find a way to pay for everything on their own. Private health insurance was available, but it was something people opted into on their own, not something provided by their employers.

The introduction of Medicare enabled many more people to have access to affordable healthcare, but earlier regulations meant that not all medical professionals were required to participate in the program.

In 1946 (after WWII), the Australian constitution was amended to ensure the prohibition of any federal law authorising medical and dental services in a manner that would result in 'any form of civil conscription' of the practitioners.[26] This meant that doctors or dentists could not be forced into working for the government.

The federal government established community health centres in the 1970s so GPs would receive the support they needed to provide health services to people at home. Community health services allowed allied health professionals to work alongside GPs to offer improved care for patients in the community. They were initially funded by a mix of federal, state/territory and local governments. However, the majority of care was still provided in hospitals. People could also have private health insurance, but the premiums were high and out of reach for many.

---

26   This amendment can be found in Section 51xxiiiA.

Medibank (the first attempt to provide a universal healthcare scheme) was established in 1975 by the Whitlam government. Medibank Private became available only to paying customers when the Liberal Party led by Malcolm Fraser was elected in 1975.

With the return of the Australian Labor Party (ALP), headed by Bob Hawke in 1983, the universal health scheme changed its name to 'Medicare'. This was considered a major social reform that aimed to produce a simple, fair and affordable insurance system that provided basic health cover for all Australians.

Medicare is now Australia's national health insurance scheme, which subsidises many medical and allied healthcare services for Australian citizens, permanent residents and those from countries which have reciprocal agreements with Australia. Medicare commenced on 1 February 1984, following the passage of the Health Legislation Amendment Act 1983.

Conservative government policies have changed the nature of funding for Medicare over the years. In 1999, the government (under John Howard) introduced the Private Health Insurance Rebate to encourage people back into the private healthcare system and reduce the pressure on the public healthcare system. Middle income families were required to pay a Medicare levy if they didn't take out private health insurance. This has had the effect of reducing the funding of the public healthcare system and further weakening the welfare state in Australia.

Private corporations have increasingly pushed into the public health sphere, which has had an overall negative impact on the quality of healthcare in Australia. The costs of private health insurance continued to increase, despite the Medicare levy and rebate, which reduced the ability of middle-class families to afford private health insurance. The big winners in this policy change have been private health insurance companies and their stakeholders.

These days, GPs and other medical specialists commonly resent the impact of the corporatisation of their patient care into what is essentially an American-style managed care system. It erodes their historical role as arbiters of the cost and degree of medical care. Although there has been an increase in the care of chronically ill patients in the community, most healthcare funding is still targeted at the acute care setting—that is, funding is aimed at curative measures rather than the improvement of the ongoing care of these patients (or prevention and management).

Australia is unique because the social services amendment of the Australian constitution is largely a product of the federal government's assumption of responsibility for health insurance after World War II, as part of a wider program of social welfare reforms. Prior to this amendment, healthcare provision was largely the responsibility of the states.

There is now a complex mix of private/public funding and state/federal funding of the Australian healthcare system. Essentially though, the federal government has required states and territories to continue to fund a large portion of the population's healthcare. This has led to distinct differences in funding arrangements across Australia's states and territories.

It is not possible here to examine these differences in detail. However, this does explain the significant differences in care provision across state and territory boundaries.

Though Australia is a large country, basic health services should be available to everyone. This is a challenge for the government. Regional and remote areas of the country are difficult to support for several reasons, a major one being the inability to attract healthcare professionals to those areas.

Without the resources that are freely available in the city—such as good schools, a variety of medical specialists and services, sporting facilities and arts communities—attracting good healthcare professionals to these areas has been an ongoing challenge for government. There have been extremely generous awards for medical practitioners willing to work in these areas.

In addition, people working in these areas must expend more time and effort to develop a relationship with their new community. Local residents are often wary of newcomers because they have experienced the extremely transitional nature of their healthcare professionals.

If a crisis occurs, then the new healthcare worker is often the only person available to manage it. It can take hours, even by plane, to get support into an area. If equipment is required, as it often is, it can take even longer. As a healthcare practitioner, therefore, you may be the only medical support for days. Emergencies can take different forms, so you have to be confident in your knowledge and experience.

From a government perspective, it is not easy to find a solution. Few healthcare professionals have the skills and temperament to handle such a responsibility, and it's difficult to convince them to make the attempt.

The health and community support landscape is continually changing: government policy is currently driving competitive tendering, which leads to different health programs being delivered by different organisations—confusing the system further and reducing its effectiveness.

Even though different states and territories have different funding streams, everyone should be able to access the same services across Australia. It is simply a matter of principle.

Acknowledgements

I would first like to acknowledge my ever-suffering husband Bruce for his ever-loving support and editing skills. He is my rock. I would also like to acknowledge my daughter, Teagan, for her uniqueness and talent for challenging my way of thinking. She is my grace.

Thank you as well to Catherine Moolenschot for her persistence and ability to keep me focused on my writing journey.

I would like to thank my publishers from Emerald Lake Books for their kindness and restraint when I took too long to reply to an email or misunderstood a request. Their patience is noted and regarded.

Gratitude goes out as well for the kindness of the people in my case studies who agreed to have their stories told (though changed slightly to maintain their confidentiality).

My own journey has been full of many stories of hope and tragedy, journeying through a system full of exceptional professionals working in a difficult and challenging environment. There have been many successes and some failures, but these professionals have always demonstrated an ongoing desire to do the right thing for those who are suffering. I thank you all. My journey with you has been amazing.

Finally, I would like to thank all of my patients who have allowed me into their life story, if ever so briefly. I walked by your side during times of fear and sorrow, illness and disability—the most vulnerable times in your lives. I wish you all well and hope that my contribution has had a positive impact.

About the Author

Anne Crawford (RN, RM, MPH, GAICD) has had a lifetime of training when it comes to how the Australian healthcare system works. She is a mother, daughter and granddaughter. She is also a nurse, midwife and public health-care expert with an in-depth knowledge of the Australian healthcare system.

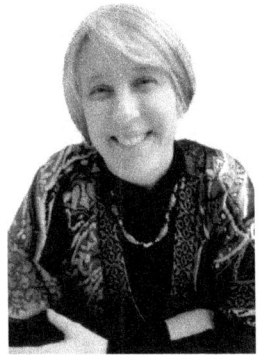

She has worked for thirty years in healthcare. Initially, as a carer, then as a professional nurse in hospitals, rehabilitation, aged care and finally in the community health setting working closely with GPs and allied health professionals. Anne now sits on the board of a community healthcare centre, private GP and dental practice. She has also set up a new and exciting business, Exploring Healthcare, providing guidance to people navigating their way through health, aged, disability and welfare services.

Anne was a primary carer for her grandmother through the aged care system at the end of her life. She also has a disabled daughter who has led her on a wonderful journey that included her need to access services in the community. Most recently, Anne sustained a traumatic injury to her eyes that changed her professional trajectory, but also meant numerous hospital visits over the past three years.

As the premier healthcare coach in Australia, she hopes to one day see many more in the healthcare industry embracing the benefits of including a healthcare coach as part of their patient care team.

> If you would like to interview Anne about healthcare coaching, or to invite her to come speak to your organization, she welcomes such inquiries and can be reached at emeraldlakebooks.com/acrawford.

For more great books, please visit us at
emeraldlakebooks.com.

EMERALD LAKE
BOOKS
Sherman, Connecticut